PAIN:
THE
ULTIMATE
MENTOR

PAIN:
THE
ULTIMATE
MENTOR

KEVIN HUNT

A CIP catalogue record for this book is available from the British Library.

For more information, email book@ultimatementor.co.uk

First paperback edition May 2023

Book cover design by Nskvsky
Typesetting by Marie Doherty

ISBN 978-1-7392925-1-5 (paperback)
ISBN 978-1-7392925-2-2 (hardback)
ISBN 978-1-7392925-0-8 (ebook)

www.ultimatementor.co.uk

Disclaimer

This book is designed to give information on various medical conditions, treatments and procedures for your personal knowledge. It is not intended to be complete or exhaustive, nor is it a substitute for the advice of your doctor. You should seek medical care promptly for any specific medical condition or problem you may have. All efforts have been made to ensure the accuracy of the information contained in this book as of the date published. I have tried to provide references as well as links to sources and further reading wherever possible. Where I refer to patients, I have anonymised those involved to ensure their privacy. I have changed details such as gender, age, occupation, circumstances and geographical location while attempting to retain the essence of their situations. Any resemblance to actual persons, living or dead, events or locales is entirely coincidental.

About the Author

KEVIN HUNT is a chartered physiotherapist with 25 years' clinical experience working with people suffering from persistent pain. He has worked with patients who have sustained multiple injuries in major accidents as well as elite athletes competing at the national and international level. He grew up in Sligo in the Republic of Ireland, completed his BSc Physiotherapy at University College Dublin, Ireland and earned a Masters in Sports & Exercise Medicine in Nottingham, UK. He runs The Spinal Physiotherapy & Sports Medicine Clinic in Cambridge, UK. He lives with his wife and two children, writes songs, plays golf and hikes mountains. This is his first book.

To Pegah, Darragh & Daniel.

Contents

Introduction

I WORK WITH PAIN. People don't come to see me because they are feeling good and want to keep things that way. They don't come to see me because they recognise that life doesn't always go to plan, and they'd like to tip the odds in their favour to reduce the risk of illness and injury down the line. They don't come to see me because they understand that we are all living longer and getting older, which increases prevalence of chronic disease and requires us to take ownership over our quality of life.

No. They come to see me because they are in pain, and they want it to stop. My job is to help them understand how pain is connected to all those issues, and that it holds the key to solving them. I help them understand pain a little differently.

Pain isn't nice, but it is much more than an unpleasant sensation. Pain is a signal to grab your attention, a protector, a guide, a call to action and a mentor. It is telling you that something needs to change. It might feel counterintuitive, but pain can help guide you in working out what those changes need to be.

Wherever you are in life – maybe you're fit and well and hoping to stay that way; maybe you're a high achiever who's used to challenging yourself; maybe you struggle to climb the stairs and get through the day; maybe you're suffering from persistent pain and feel like you've tried everything already – understanding how pain works, how it is trying to help you improve your quality of life, is what I do. You don't need to fear pain, but you do have to recognise that it is there for a reason. It's just not necessarily the reason you thought it was.

Imagine waking up tomorrow morning in a city you've never heard of, surrounded by faces you don't recognise and a language you don't understand, with no money, food or shelter, and no sense of where you are.

It would be hugely stressful, potentially overwhelming. You would learn a lot about your own strengths and weaknesses, and you would encounter both success and failure in attempting to build a usable map of this new land you find yourself in. You might look for allies or try to protect yourself from predators. You would discover how robust and resilient you are in attempting to chart a course between order and chaos.

An experienced observer who understands the world you are in would be invaluable in such a situation. They could help evaluate the decisions you make. They would be able to see if you were heading to the right part of town, associating with people who were helpful or harmful. They would be able to see if you were getting in over your head or setting your sights too low.

When you are born, you have no idea about the world you enter. You have to learn to orientate yourself, develop skills and navigate a path through life. An observer or mentor who understands that would be a hugely helpful ally. The good news is we all have such a mentor within us. That mentor is the pain system. Pain is the ultimate protector. It will help guide you if you are willing to listen, but you need to understand how it works.

Your developing nervous system adapts and responds to the environment you grow up in, the experiences you have and the people you meet, the support or neglect you receive. It's a plastic system that changes and learns, but it also needs to be updated regularly.

How you see the world shapes the circuits and systems in your brain. Your body uses chemical messengers called neurotransmitters to stimulate these systems positively or negatively; in turn, they continue to adapt and respond. These neurotransmitters are governed by the life you live – and the life you live is governed by such systems. The challenge is how to live in a way that builds the best system for you: to do that, you need a guide that understands the world you are in and can help you navigate it. That is the job of the pain system.

All too often I hear people try to separate pain into physical or emotional pain. I see people with persistent pain wondering if they are simply imagining their pain, if it is "all in the mind". Pain is pain. Experiencing pain is a function of being human, and there are many factors that influence this experience. Factors that turn the pain up and factors that turn it down. Most of these are within your control, and your choices, behaviours and understanding of such things matter more than you realise.

Conventionally, medical science distinguishes between three types of pain.

Nociceptive pain occurs when the nociceptive fibres – essentially the body's inbuilt threat detectors – get activated in acute tissue trauma, such as a fracture, an arthritis flare-up or a torn muscle, ligament or tendon. In turn this activates your immune system and a local inflammatory response to stimulate healing. The time frame for this type of pain is less than three months. For such classic "injury", pain medications can help as they influence the nociceptive system.

Neuropathic pain results from nerve damage, such as after surgery where a nerve may have been cut; when the nervous system is injured or diseased, such as in a spinal cord lesion, multiple sclerosis or diabetes; or when it is damaged by drug or alcohol abuse. Medication can help but can't necessarily provide lasting relief.

Nociplastic pain is the main source of persistent pain and pain flare-ups. It happens when the central nervous system of the brain and spinal cord gets sensitised. Pain medications do not work on this system.

Pain is described as persistent when it lasts for more than three months and is no longer primarily driven by nociception. Persistent pain doesn't mean being in pain all the time, although it might feel that way. Sometimes pain takes the form of regular headaches or a classic "bad back" that goes at the most inconvenient times. Nociplastic pain is involved in these scenarios, and it is influenced – as you will discover – by your lifestyle, your mindset and the information you are exposed to along the way. It is absolutely not "all in your mind".

The good news is that the answer to nociplastic pain doesn't lie in medications, injections and operations. If you're reading this book, you may well have already discovered that for yourself. Instead, the answer lies in understanding the detail of the six essential aspects of your lifestyle and how much they affect your well-being. Together these make up what I call your health hexagon:

Physical life	Emotional life
Mental life	Sleep
Spiritual life	Diet

There is nothing radically new there, and you may already believe that you know all you need to know about each of these elements and how they function within your lifestyle. What you may not realise is that nociplastic pain is not just an irritation to be endured or medicated away. (That simply won't work for this type of pain anyway.) It is acting as a mentor to guide you when you are getting all or any of these elements wrong.

Understanding how all this works and why it matters will improve anyone's quality of life. If you suffer from persistent pain, then it just might allow you to change your pain sensitivity and achieve your goals without it being such a painful experience along the way. If you haven't experienced persistent pain, you will still benefit: as the old adage goes, prevention is better than cure.

Persistent pain doesn't always fit neatly into one category. Most persistent pain problems I see in clinic are of a mixed nature. There will be some nociceptive pain initially, following an injury or a flare-up of a condition such as arthritis, and sometimes underlying nociplastic pain if the problem has gone on longer than three months. If I see someone with a first-time acute injury (less than six weeks old), I try to help them avoid turning that injury into a persistent pain problem by helping them understand the significance of some of the topics we will explore in this book. If they are primarily suffering from nociplastic pain, then I focus on helping them see the connection between that pain and the factors in their life that may be aggravating or amplifying it. This is about making structural, not just mindset, change.

My purpose with this book is to help you understand how pain works so that you can see how it is trying to guide you through building a better lifestyle. Sometimes it protects you from outside influence; sometimes it is trying to protect you from yourself. In whatever form it takes, pain is there to grab your attention, and how you deal with it will affect how your system responds in the future.

In an ideal world, you'd give enough attention to each element of your hexagon. The trouble is most of us don't live in an ideal world. Let's say you're going through a difficult period at work. You work longer hours, trying to meet a deadline or get something done, doubling down on your efforts to control the stress. As a result you haven't exercised for a while, your diet isn't great, you can't remember the last time you had a decent night's sleep, you've neglected close relationships and you haven't switched off for ages. You're tired, snappy and frustrated that those around you don't realise how hard you are working. On top of that perhaps you're now getting some pain: headaches, say, or your back goes. It's a familiar story – and all too predictable for many of us.

Maybe work has had to take a back seat while you care for a family member. Perhaps you're hitting the gym five times a week, hoping that losing some weight will make everything OK. Perhaps you're feeling burnt out from a high-flying job in the city, the perks no longer providing the satisfaction they once did, and thinking about a major life U-turn in a quest for greater purpose.

So, things are out of balance. What happens now when something unexpected occurs, which it inevitably will from time to time? A bereavement, redundancy, financial uncertainty, health crisis, work disaster, relationship turbulence, the boiler breaking down just as the in-laws arrive for Christmas?

Modern life is complex, but deep down we are still primitive animals with basic needs. We all understand that some form of balance is necessary in life. Too much of anything, good or bad, isn't helpful or healthy. When that knock on the door comes, which it inevitably will, you want to be able to deal with whatever comes your way rather than already feeling depleted and overwhelmed.

When I talk about balance, you might think of work-life balance and picture a see-saw, with work on one side and life on the other. But this clearly gives work a heavier weighting against all the other elements of life. I prefer to think about balance as more of a hexagonal merry-go-round. To keep that merry-go-round moving, you need to get the correct weighting in the various parts of your life. That's not necessarily equal, but enough in each element for the stage of life you are at.

I'll be talking a lot throughout the book about the consequences of a pro-inflammatory lifestyle. What do I mean by that? Inflammation is a necessary part of your body's defence systems against illness, injury and disease. Anything that threatens the body will ignite an inflammatory response in some way. If you are exposed to a virus, your immune system defends itself with an inflammatory response. If you cut your skin, tear a muscle or fracture a bone, your body's inflammatory response system kick-starts the healing process. When the response is appropriate, this is very helpful. However, some medical conditions generate too strong an inflammatory reaction, for instance rheumatoid arthritis or Crohn's disease, and they need careful treatment to manage inflammation.

Separate from such medical conditions, a pro-inflammatory life is anything that consistently acts as a perceived threat to the body and so provokes an inflammatory response. That might include lifestyle factors such as eating unhealthily, not getting enough rest, being under psychological stress or engaging in risk-taking behaviours. Of course, some exposure to threat is healthy, but we're talking here about consistency over a period of time. There might not be any obvious impact on your body or life initially, but over time you can end up living with a low-level drip, drip, drip of stress that is unsustainable in the long run. Your body becomes a chronic inflammatory environment, which has implications for your health and well-being, as you will discover.

Pro-inflammatory lifestyle factors have been shown to contribute to the rise in chronic health conditions such as heart disease, type 2 diabetes, arthritis, autoimmune conditions and musculoskeletal conditions. You might not realise your lifestyle is why you are experiencing pain – it might seem more intuitive to blame it on an apparent physical cause, like "sleeping wrong" or "stretching weirdly". By the end of this book, I hope I'll have helped you see the bigger picture – to understand how the way you live and the choices you make shape the way you feel. Just as certain ways of living can promote inflammation, choosing to do things differently can reduce inflammation and reduce the impact and risk of illness, injury and disease.

In my clinical practice over the last 25 years, I have been privileged to treat a wide variety of people, from Olympic athletes to weekend warriors and those struggling to climb a flight of stairs. I have worked with celebrated academics and people who are illiterate. I have helped clients who struggle to get a job and CEOs of companies employing thousands of people. My patients range in age from 8 to 96 and include consultant physicians, surgeons, nurses, musicians, artists, builders, bakers, soldiers and sailors.

Besides coming to see me for help with pain, they all have one thing in common. They all needed help organising their hexagon and a better understanding of how pain can be a helpful guide, rather than fighting or fearing it.

Why does any of this matter, especially if you are not suffering from persistent pain? A systematic review and meta-analysis published in the *British Medical Journal* in 2016 estimated that one-third to one-half of Britons suffered from chronic/persistent pain and anticipated this number to grow.[1] Similar results are seen in other countries – globally an estimated 1.9 billion people suffer from recurrent tension-type headache alone.[2] The consensus within the area of managing persistent pain is that strategies need to take into account the biological, psychological, sociodemographic and lifestyle factors that influence pain. The health hexagon provides some structure to this while also recognising pain as a system that helps us self-regulate and alerts us when we are drifting into chaos.

Using stories from patients I have treated, I will help you understand how your biochemistry and nervous system behave in each of the six essential elements of your health hexagon. I will explain how the pain pathway works, how your brain processes such things and how stress and lifestyle influence it, and I'll offer some steps to recalibrate your pain system. You can choose whether to dig deeper into the science or to take the general principles I offer you and move on.

It's common to get confused, annoyed, angry and frustrated with persistent pain. That's understandable, but it doesn't help. Instead I hope that by the end of this book you will see how pain, although a blunt tool, is trying to guide and mentor you.

Let's begin.

CHAPTER 1

The Purpose of Pain

I TREAT PEOPLE with persistent pain. People whose pain is preventing them from doing the things they want to do. The things that will give them fulfilment and satisfaction in life. People who have failed to improve with time. People who get frequent flare-ups of pain that don't make sense, or they try to make sense of them in a way that only makes things worse. People who have tried all sorts of treatments and therapies and myths and potions and often failed surgeries. The health hexagon is a way for them to recalibrate their system. To recalibrate, you need to understand how pain works, what it's trying to do and why we sometimes misunderstand its purpose.

Most of us grow up believing that pain means damage and we can only experience pain if we have injured ourselves, broken a bone or done something "wrong". It's not that simple. Hurt and harm are not the same.

Pain is there to guide you, alert you to potential danger, so you consider your actions before repeating them. Pain remembers past events, using them to predict future possibilities. It's remarkable. It's like a supercomputer storing all the data you have encountered in your entire life for future reference, not to mention the circuity you've inherited from previous generations and the fine-tuning of these systems throughout the evolution of our species. These circuits, in part inherited, also develop throughout your lifetime like software updates. Some circuits become stronger than others, some need to be relearned, some need to be upgraded and some crash the system. Pain learns – and that is both the beauty of the system and the potential problem.

We used to use the term "chronic pain" when talking about pain that went on longer than three months, but over time the definition of chronic pain became blurred. For some people chronic meant forever. For some chronic meant dull, and for others it meant severe. The term "persistent pain" is now widely used instead. As I said in the introduction, this is essentially pain that lasts longer than three months.[1,2] On the whole, tissues heal in about three months – that covers muscles, ligaments, tendons, skin, bone. Beyond three months, pain is no longer a reliable measure of tissue harm or tissue damage.

This is not to suggest that any pain beyond three months is somehow imagined or unnecessary. All pain is real. It's just that it is not a reliable indicator of harm or damage. We are not talking about acute pain scenarios such as cutting yourself or dislocating your shoulder, or in disease processes like rheumatoid arthritis, although some of the principles still apply. We also are not talking about cancer-related pain. That's a separate thing entirely and not within the scope of this book. We are talking about persistent pain that continues beyond three months after the structure has healed or where there is no obvious damage in the first place.

Consider it this way. Let's say you broke your ankle. You've been put in a boot to immobilise the ankle for two months to allow the bones to knit together. All is healing well, and at the two-month mark the X-rays are satisfactory, showing that the alignment of the bones are good, the fracture site is filling in nicely and it's safe to take off the boot and start rehabilitating. Does this mean you would now expect to be pain-free? Of course not. You haven't moved your ankle for two months and there will be a lot of muscle wastage and stiffness. Would you expect it to be painful to start moving that foot? Yes. Do you think it would be painful to start taking some small steps? Absolutely. Does it mean you shouldn't even try to take a step until you are pain-free? No, that's not going to work. To rehabilitate you need to start doing something. Your physiotherapist will guide you through that process and help you work with your pain.

As you start to walk on it again, it will be painful. Does that mean you are breaking your ankle again? It might feel like that to begin with, but this is not the case. By 12 weeks, if all is going well with your rehabilitation, things will be more comfortable. You might even be off your crutches and fully weight-bearing. The bones won't yet be skeletally mature, as turning fresh bone after a fracture into mature bone takes about a year, but in this scenario you should be strong enough at three months to increase the rehab. At this point the pain is no longer a reliable indicator of tissue damage. You are now into persistent pain territory. You are not breaking the bone every time you get pain, but you're still having a pain experience. Now you start to recalibrate your pain system as your rehab progresses.

This might all seem a bit obvious with a broken bone. What about when the injury or pain isn't so clear to begin with? Take back pain, neck pain or knee pain that goes on for months, maybe even years, without you knowing why it started in the first place. What is the role of pain then?

I like to consider pain like parking sensors in a car. When you hear those beeps for the first time, chances are you slammed on

3

the brakes, anxious you were about to hit something. Once you calmed down and surveyed the area, you realised you had some space, and you eased your way along, allowing the parking sensors to guide you and help you change direction as required. In time, you learned to understand what the beeps meant and how much space you had to work with.

We used to think that pain could only be produced when we did damage. In the car analogy this is when you hit the wall. In reality, and with persistent pain in particular, pain is more like the parking sensors guiding and warning you before you hit the wall. They are trying to grab your attention to prevent you from doing harm. The challenge is accepting and understanding this – and realising that in many circumstances the persistent pain parking sensors are more sensitised than they need to be. This book will help you understand how to recalibrate them to an appropriate level. If we don't understand the role of pain, we slam on the brakes too heavily and end up terrified of moving altogether.

With certain pains or parts of your body, this is fairly easy to understand. With a headache, you may let the pain guide you. Maybe you need an early night, maybe you need more fluid or something to eat. Maybe you need glasses. You don't panic or catastrophise. In this scenario you have a sense of your parking sensors' sensitivity and you let the sensors guide you in making a decision, such as getting more sleep.

What if you get pain in a part of your body that you are not familiar with or a flare-up while you're doing something that's never caused pain before? That might feel a bit like hiring a holiday car in the airport rather than driving your own, familiar car. You have to go through the whole recalibration process again to get a sense of how much room these parking sensors give you in comparison to your car's sensors. If you don't understand what the sensors are trying to do, you end up stuck in the car park.

Of course, coping with persistent pain isn't quite the same as parking a car. It's not so easy to "see" how much space you have to play with. But too often persistent pain stops you from doing what will help you feel better in the long run. This in turn leads your pain system to becoming more sensitised; your parking sensors start beeping even sooner than before, and the cycle continues.

The thing about persistent pain is that everyone with persistent pain has pain-free moments. They don't always recognise them. But I promise you, take the time to observe and you will see that there are moments without pain. Because there are moments without pain, there are things that turn the pain up and things that turn the pain down. They just won't necessarily be what you think they are.

Those pain-free moments can also be days, weeks, months or even years. Persistent pain can cover a lifetime. Perhaps you don't even realise you have a persistent pain problem. Maybe you have a "bad back" that mysteriously "goes" every so often. You have long periods of it being fine and then randomly it goes. You've convinced yourself – or someone else has tried to convince you – that there was a problem, maybe your pelvis was "out of line", but they've manipulated it back into place now, until the next time it goes.

I deal with serious injuries daily. I've seen what a pelvis out of line looks like, and you don't do it putting your socks on. Your back may go into a real spasm after a minor insult because your stress response system, the hypothalamic-pituitary-adrenal axis, was already stimulated by a pro-inflammatory lifestyle, leading to your inflammatory system becoming more aggressive than necessary and generating a guarding spasm response. That can be painful of course, but your spine is not "out of line". But if you're convinced that this is what has happened and your parking sensors are beeping, naturally you will be afraid to move or at best move extremely cautiously – and everything will look like a threat. You're more likely to stop doing all the things that are good for your hexagon – and as a result the pain will intensify.

Pain is unique. There is no average, and the next chapters are going to unravel the pain pathway to help you make sense of it. Let's start with the story of a jockey whose horse fell on him. That's got to be painful. Hasn't it?

CHAPTER 2

The Context of Pain

THE PHONE LINE RECEPTION wasn't great, but I could just make out the words against the background noise of what I suspect was motorway traffic.

"I think I've broken my ankle."

Phone calls like this are not uncommon in my world. Dealing with the trials and tribulations of working jockeys has taught me a lot about pain. No distress, no panic in this man's voice, just a hint of frustration about the possible disruption to his day.

"What makes you think your ankle's broken?" I ask.

"Well, my foot was pointing the wrong way."

"Fair enough." I've heard this sort of thing more than once. "Tell me what happened."

"I was riding out this morning, but the horse wasn't sound, so I pulled up. I was walking him back to the yard and he slipped and pulled me down and landed on my leg. I heard a crack and my foot was pointing the wrong way."

"OK, what did you do then?"

"I sort of pulled it a bit and wiggled it and it seems OK now."

"Is it painful?" I know that this won't necessarily help me come to a decision, but it seems polite to ask under the circumstances.

"Not really."

"Could you walk on it straight away?"

"I was a bit lame but yeah, I walked back to the yard. It was only about two hundred metres though. Do you think it's broken?"

"Are you driving right now?" I was fairly confident I already knew the answer.

"Yeah, but it's OK, it's my left ankle and I'm driving an automatic. Do you think you could strap it up or something? I'm riding at Lingfield this evening."

"I think you should drive to A&E," I say matter of factly.

"Really?" comes the knowingly resigned retort. He wouldn't have called if he was expecting anything else. Deep down he knew things weren't right, but he needed to hear that he wasn't wasting everyone's time.

"Really. Your foot was pointing the wrong way. That's a fairly strong indication you've broken something."

Silence.

"What about Lingfield this evening?" he asks optimistically.

"Let's wait and see what the hospital says first. Oh, and by the way: insist they X-ray you."

"What do you mean?" he asks, puzzled. I can sense his reluctance. The thought of retelling the tale in A&E, having to wait with the screamers, the coughers, the battle-axe receptionist, the endless questions: "Was it a big horse? Was it a fast horse? Any tips? Do you know Frankie?"

"When you walk in there in your jodhpurs and boots," I explain, "without any obvious signs of pain or distress, they're probably going to send you on your way without an X-ray. You need to tell them that you must have an X-ray. Don't leave without one. Let me know how you get on."

A few hours later he calls back.

"So, what's the story?" I ask.

"Yeah, it's broken. They're operating on me in a couple of hours."

"Did you have much hassle in A&E?"

"They were a bit snotty. Didn't think much was wrong with me as I could walk on it. I think they only X-rayed me to get me out of there. They were quite surprised it was as badly broken as it was. No Lingfield tonight."

How can someone have a horse land on them and then walk into A&E as cool as a cucumber? Well, it's partly to do with context. When a jockey comes off a horse or the horse rolls on top of them, a broken ankle is a good result. Of course they will be frustrated about missing work while they recover, and likely anxious about whether someone else will take their place while they're injured. But in horse racing, anything short of being paralysed is a good result. Breaking your ankle is almost something of a relief by comparison. It's a common injury in this world, and no one has lost their career as a result.

In this context, a broken ankle is a nuisance but not the end of the world – and the jockey's experience of the pain will not be as severe as it might be for a ballerina with a broken ankle. In ballet, a broken ankle is of far greater consequence. It could end a dancer's career. This could be devastating, and the pain experience will likely be far greater.

It's easy to think that the jockey has a higher pain threshold than the ballerina, but this is not the case. No doubt that same ballerina would be capable of putting up with more discomfort in her toes from years and years of being *en pointe* than the jockey could tolerate. I'm also pretty sure, from direct experience, that the jockey who is capable of walking on a broken ankle after falling off a horse would be much more distressed if he woke up one morning with a pain in his foot for no apparent reason. Without an obvious reason, like a fall, he might worry that it indicated a serious problem, such as the onset of arthritis, which would jeopardise his career. For the rest of us, getting out of bed with a sore foot one random morning is nothing much to worry about. Chances are we would give it a day or two to see if it disappeared before getting too animated. The ballerina meanwhile is likely used to waking up with painful feet most days and takes it as part of the territory.

So, the circumstances in which you experience pain affect how you feel that pain. The idea that you have either a high or a low pain threshold is not helpful here. In fact, even within your body, you may experience pain differently depending on context. Studies have shown that right-handed professional violinists have higher pain sensitivity in their left hand than in their right hand.[1] Think about this. The same individual has a different pain tolerance for the same body part on different sides. Why?

The left hand is the one that manipulates the strings. As a right-handed violinist, you could injure your right hand, maybe even lose a finger or two, and still theoretically manage to work a bow; but any injury to the fingers of your left hand could be catastrophic. Over time your body learns to treat the left hand with greater care while the pathways that control such things become more sensitive on the left than on the right. Even though the dominant hand is statistically more likely to get injured, the body protects the left hand more carefully.

Let's take a closer look at how the pain pathway works.

Black box feeling

To experience anything, you go through three stages. The first is sensory information. This is where one or more of your senses are stimulated: sight, sound, smell, taste, touch and a sixth sense that is understood as a general sense of awareness, sometimes referred to as blindsight. Next, these messages are filtered through stored data, which is everything you have taken from past experiences, belief systems, sensitivity to threat, personality traits and so on. Various regions of your brain will negotiate with each other during this stage. Once your brain has filtered the incoming messages, you get predicted data. This is what your brain decides is the appropriate response, and that is what you experience. The pain pathway is also made up of these three stages, and each stage can be influenced by how you organise your health hexagon.

When you touch something, your brain will attach some emotional relevance to it. For example, when you touch a soft blanket, your brain might think "fluffy like a teddy bear". The experience you have on touching that object might then be classified as soft, comforting, safe. Now imagine placing your hand inside a box to feel for unknown objects while blindfolded. You feel something slightly soft, a little warm. Someone tells you there is nothing dangerous in the box, so you explore a little more. Someone else tells you there are several objects in there, one of which is a rat. Suddenly your experience changes. Unless you love rats, you are likely to feel creeped out. Perhaps your heart starts racing, you breathe quickly, you tense your muscles and you feel a strong urge to withdraw your hand. It's the same sensory stimulus but the experience is very different.

This is how the body works. We give greater weight to the negative information (there is a rat in there) than the positive information (there's nothing dangerous in there) due to the filtering process by certain parts of the brain, which are trying to protect us from harm.

Information and how you understand it matters. Your brain's filtering system relies on it. Say someone in a position of authority tells you that your spine is out of line. That will influence what you feel and how you react. You might trust the individual who tells you that the box is safe, but even so your limbic system (the brain's emotional centre) will most likely give the balance of power to the negative information that it is unsafe, and your prefrontal cortex (the executive centre of the brain responsible for a higher level of thinking) will have to work harder to negotiate with the limbic system. You might use your prefrontal cortex to consider the consequences of removing your hand from the box and what that might mean for your status in that situation. Will you look weak for removing it? Will this look like you don't really trust your friend? You might attempt to use top-down control to regulate your emotional and visceral responses, such as consciously taking slow, deep breaths, or reminding yourself that you can do this, and no one is trying to harm you.

Once your brain has processed incoming sensory stimuli and filtered them through context, consequences, risk and reward, it will activate other regions to respond accordingly. This is the predicted data. You will trigger an emotional response; your autonomic nervous system will instruct your endocrine system to react by releasing hormones into the bloodstream; and your organs will react accordingly. Your heart rate, blood pressure, respiratory rate, and body temperature will be instructed as to what they should do. Blood flow will decrease in certain areas of the body and increase in others, depending on perceived need. All of this is happening in real time and your brain will remember these circumstances, collecting more information to use as stored data for the future.

Putting your hand in that box is not as simple as merely feeling what's inside. You have to decide how you will interact with the contents and how that experience will affect you. When you do, this will in part influence what happens next as well as how you behave in a similar situation in the future. You will be reinforcing some pathways that will fire automatically, and updating stored data to help you make decisions in the future. You do this all the time, often without paying attention to what you are doing or why you behaved the way you did. This is particularly true when it comes to persistent pain.

Let's go on a journey through the pain pathway.

CHAPTER 3

The Sensory Bus Ride

YOUR NERVOUS SYSTEM has many checks and balances that allow you to interact with the world around you. It needs a way of delivering outside information to your internal environment so you can react, make decisions and run on autopilot to some degree. You need a system that allows you to be aware of what's salient and not distracted by what isn't. Think of it this way. If you put on a pair of gloves, you feel the sensation of those gloves interacting with your skin. That's good. You don't need to feel that sensation constantly though. That might distract you from other things that could be more important and necessary for survival. So after a while the sensory messages from the gloves on your skin can be filtered out or ignored. Your body is constantly having to prioritise.

The first time you drive somewhere, you have to concentrate hard to figure out where you are going, pay attention to landmarks en route, calculate how much time it will take to get there and estimate what extra time you may need to allow in case of traffic or unforeseen circumstances. If you're making the journey by bus, you might need to work out the timetable and where you need to change buses or the cost of a ticket. But if you repeat that journey regularly, it becomes so routine that you may often have no memory of making it on a particular occasion.

At some level you were paying attention – you didn't crash – but your brain was doing this for you automatically. Once a process becomes automatic, unless something unusual happens the chances are you don't really remember it. If you had to consciously process every single detail, every single time, you wouldn't get much done. This whole process is how the brain learns and builds systems of information. When you repeat something again and again, the nervous system builds a pathway to process that piece of data. The more you use that pathway, the stronger or more efficient it gets. It starts to become almost like a reflex. This is how you develop expertise in anything. An athlete repeating the same action again and again develops stronger pathways that perform that action. The nerves delivering the messages travel faster than they would for an amateur performing the same action who has spent less time practising it.[1]

This is true of things that are good for you and not so good for you. If you repeat the same behaviours time and time again, you can be building good processes as well as bad. The great thing about the nervous system is that it is plastic: it can adapt and rewrite information or create new pathways to replace existing ones. You can break bad habits, change your attitude towards something or alter how you deal with certain situations. You can learn and relearn, if you are willing to do so.

To explain how this works in the pain pathway, I am going to use the analogy of a bus journey. It's not a perfect analogy by any means, but I think it gets the point across.

To understand how your body processes pain, we first need to look at how potentially dangerous signals make their way to the brain to be processed. Your body needs a system to decide whether a message is "safe" or "potentially dangerous". In time, from a pain point of view, it can ignore the safe signals and alert you only to the potentially dangerous ones. You start running on autopilot unless something needs to grab your attention. To do this, your brain uses sensory detectors called nociceptors. These sensory threat detectors line the surfaces of your body such as the skin (as well as other body parts such as the gut, muscles and bones) and act as the interface between your external (somatic) and internal (autonomic) environments. They respond to potentially damaging stimuli by sending "possible threat" signals to the spinal cord, which are then relayed to the brain. If deemed appropriate, the result will be that you experience pain.

Nociception and *pain* are not interchangeable terms: you can have a pain experience without stimulating nociceptive fibres, and you can stimulate nociceptive fibres without getting a pain experience. This will become clearer as you learn more about the pain pathway. The nociceptors let the central nervous system know that there is a potentially dangerous stimulus nearby, not that it is definitely dangerous. Think of putting your hand over a candle flame to see how long you can keep it there. Your thermal nociceptors will be activated to make the central nervous system aware of a potentially dangerous input coming from outside, but the degree of your pain experience will be determined later by your brain's filtering system.

Your body contains various other kinds of receptors to detect changes in external stimuli. Each of these detectors has a different physical shape and is stimulated by different things such as temperature or pressure. Once stimulated the sensor sends signals into the central nervous system at different frequencies – a bit like Morse code – to indicate that this is a pressure sensor signal rather than a temperature signal. Of course, both could be stimulated

17

at the same time, so your brain needs to understand what each signal means in order to process them.

When you think of nerves, you might imagine hair-like electric cables running around your body. At their tiniest they are thread-like, but nerves are often much bigger than you realise. The sciatic nerve runs down your leg from your spine and is as thick as your thumb in places. It is involved in sensory and motor function for certain parts of the leg, determining what you feel and how you move. You can think of nerves like fibre optic cables delivering data from the sensory elements of the peripheral nervous system into the central nervous system (brain and spinal cord) where it is processed, and then applying that processing to deliver an experience or action to the body. You feel yourself putting on your socks – that's sensory. You decide you need to get to the other side of the room, so you walk – that's motor. Your nervous system does this.

When you touch something, you activate several sensors on your skin: pressure sensors, temperature receptors, chemoreceptors, voltage receptors. Each sends a signal along a first-order neuron from the skin into the dorsal horn of the spinal cord (an intermediary processing centre), delivering information from the outside world to your central nervous system. This is the first of many synapses on the journey of that touch. A synapse is where a neuron communicates with another neuron to transmit a message.

Going back to the bus analogy, a neuron is like a bus carrying a passenger (the stimulus) along the road until it reaches the end of its route. In this scenario the route, the neuron, runs from the skin to the dorsal horn of the spinal cord. The passenger now needs to change buses to travel on a second-order neuron that will take it from the dorsal horn of the spinal cord up to the brain.

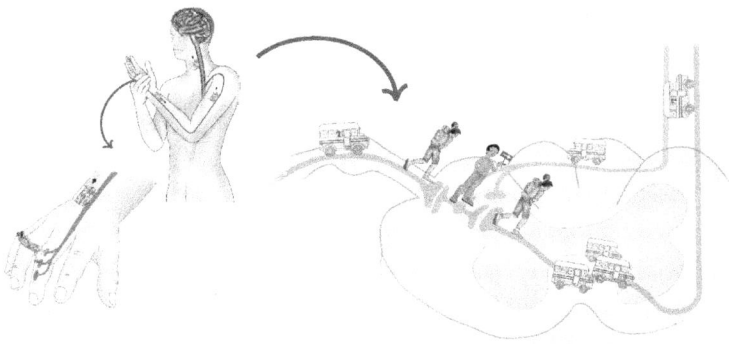

Figure 1: The Sensory Bus Ride

Activation of a nociceptive sensor sets a passenger (the stimulus) on a bus ride along the first-order neuron to the dorsal horn of the spinal cord. Within the spinal cord the passenger communicates with the traffic controller (the astrocyte) for permission to change buses (synapse). The passenger takes a waiting bus to deliver that message to the brain via a second-order neuron.

This happens at the synapse – similar to a bus terminus. The passenger needs a system that allows them to change buses. This is where neurotransmitters come in. These are the tickets that grant access or permission to get on the next bus. Armed with a ticket (neurotransmitter), the passenger leaves the first bus and walks across the terminus to find the right bus for the next part of the journey. That all seems simple so far, right?

To complicate things a little, the synapse or bus terminus is usually not just one neuron meeting another neuron. It's more like one neuron communicating with potentially 1,000 different neurons.[2] That's 1,000 different buses to choose from. That's why the passenger needs a system of communication to figure out the correct bus to take. At different parts of the nervous system, the potential number of postsynaptic neurons (buses) can be as many as 100,000. That's a lot of information to process. And this isn't just happening in one place at one time. Your senses are constantly receiving tens of thousands of stimuli all over your body: these "buses" are delivering passengers all over the network, up and down the entire length of the spinal cord all the time.

Why so many buses? Because there are many possible pieces of information that need to be processed. Each time you do something, you need to use an existing pathway or establish a new one that you can then learn for future reference. Touching something isn't just a matter of touching something. Your nervous system needs a way to figure out if that thing is hard, soft, bumpy, fluffy, smooth, rough, sharp, dull, warm, tepid, hot, cold, slimy, moist, dry, old, new, shiny, expensive, cheap or brittle. Any number of pieces of data need to be considered, and it's not just your skin sensors contributing to the decision-making process. Your eyes are capturing data and sending those data into the system too, as are your ears: What shape is it? What colour is it? Is it squeaky? Is it crunchy? Does it smell? All these pieces of data need a specific pathway to follow so you have the information you need to assess a stimulus and hence an impressive number of postsynaptic neurons to choose from to deliver the various pieces of data your brain needs to figure out what to do in response.

So that thing you touched has more than likely started a whole load of buses on their journey, armed with different pieces of information all destined for different parts of the nervous system to give the brain – or command centre – the data it requires to orientate yourself in the world every moment of every day. As so many messages are being processed, you need a lot of roads to keep the system flowing. Almost every synapse in the central nervous system is like a major bus terminus in a metropolis. On top of that there are an estimated 86 billion neurons in the brain, each with potentially 7 to 10,000 synapses.[3] At this point we're still talking about data. Your brain has to process each piece and decide what it is before it gets converted into a sensation. This information is travelling at up to 275 mph and zips around the system very fast indeed.[4] Is it any wonder things get confused from time to time? In such a system it's easy to take the wrong bus occasionally.

If you have a spinal cord injury, any incoming messages below the level of the spinal cord lesion won't be able to travel up to the brain as they can't travel past the site of the injury and therefore a sensation can't be realised. Trauma can occur to the tissues below the spinal cord injury, but you won't feel them, demonstrating that pain doesn't happen at the site of the injury. To generate a pain sensation, your brain must decide what's going on with the information it receives.

21

Similarly, pain can occur in an area even when there is no trauma to the tissues. Phantom limb pain is a good example of the brain generating a pain sensation in tissue that isn't there. The pain is very real indeed, but the cause is not always obvious. As I said earlier, you can stimulate nociceptive fibres and not experience pain; and you can experience pain without stimulating nociceptive fibres. Going back to my jockey, he stimulated a whole load of nociceptive fibres in breaking his ankle, but his pain experience wasn't universal. There is more to the pain experience than just nociception. So why are these fibres necessary? Well, they have a very important function. They provide information to help your body decide if something is safe or potentially dangerous.

Every sensory encounter you have is continuously being processed, whether you are consciously aware of it or not. There is so much going on within your nervous system all the time. To prevent you from exploding under such an assault to the senses, the nociceptors have a threshold at which they will be activated. For example, when it comes to temperature, in normal circumstances the nociceptive thermoreceptors will be activated only at temperatures below 18 degrees C or above 25 degrees C.[5,6] If you touch something between 19 degrees and 24 degrees, they won't react. You'll still feel that temperature from other sensory thermoreceptors, just not nociceptive ones. If, however, you touch something that is 17 degrees or 26 degrees, you will stimulate these nociceptive thermoreceptors and your brain will get some sensory data to help it work out whether your environment is getting potentially too cold or too hot. It will use this information – among many other pieces of data – to come up with a response.

Going back to the example of the candle flame, when you put your hand above the flame initially, you won't feel much. Only as the temperature goes up and reaches the threshold at which the nociceptive fibres get stimulated does your central nervous system get alerted that things are getting hot. In response to a potential danger your body acts to make you feel uncomfortable, maybe in pain, so you withdraw your hand. The pain doesn't happen *because* you've burned yourself: it's trying to prevent you from burning yourself.

To complicate things a little further, the threshold at which your nociceptive fibres are activated is also influenced by inflammation.[7] In the presence of inflammation, the nociceptive fibres become easier to stimulate. There is a good reason for this when it comes to injury: to make you more sensitive so that you can protect the injured area. If you sprain your ankle, the ligament needs time to heal. Making your leg sensitive to pressure and stretch means you will rest the area.

The nociceptive sensors in the ligament itself will generate peripheral pain: they will contribute to producing a pain response when stimulated locally, such as when you touch, stretch or move the affected area. To protect the damaged ankle ligament, which is only a couple of centimetres long, the pain system will also recruit the surrounding area (the rest of the foot) to become tender and sensitive. This creates a zone of sensitivity around the injured part. Your little toe will be painful after you've sprained your ankle, but you haven't damaged the little toe itself. It becomes sensitive so that if anything comes near your foot, you'll react and protect the whole foot to keep safe the injured part. The pain system does this through the central nervous system in the spinal cord and this is called pain central sensitisation.[8] The synapses in the spinal cord start to make connections locally so that messages coming from neurons from the injured tissue and areas around it get treated as potentially dangerous.

Typically, as tissues heal and an injury gets better, the region of pain shrinks and the centralisation element diminishes. Your ligament may be locally tender but the rest of the foot returns to normal, allowing you to put more weight on it and start rehabilitating the structure. You start trusting that you can do more with the injured part as part of your recovery.

Unfortunately, in some cases the centralised pain system can become so good at protecting the area that the pain persists even when it is no longer helpful or necessary as an indicator of damage.[9] Three months after an injury, pain is no longer a reliable indicator of harm or damage. It doesn't mean that you are not experiencing pain. You may well be, but not necessarily for the reasons you think. The ligament has more than likely healed structurally, but the pain system is staying sensitised for a variety of reasons that will become clearer as you progress through this book. It continues to be painful, but this is now no longer a true indicator of harm or damage. This is nociplastic pain, as mentioned in the introduction.

A pro-inflammatory lifestyle can lead the nociceptors to become more sensitive. They then send signals into the central nervous system more readily, which can be filtered as a threat. The result is your body creates a pain experience when no tissue damage has occurred. This is not uncommon in persistent pain.[10] The pain is real, but the structure isn't necessarily damaged.

As mentioned, neurotransmitters are required to pass the message from the first-order neuron to the second-order neuron in the synapse at the dorsal horn of the spinal cord. (They are also involved in the messaging system within the brain.) If the correct neurotransmitters arrive at the postsynaptic neuron (second bus) and they have the appropriate receptor (valid ticket), then the neuron will carry the message along. If the neurotransmitter does not get released (no ticket purchased for the next bus) or does not find an appropriate receptor at the other end of the terminus (misses the bus), then the message dies. You will see that your lifestyle choices have a significant impact on the neurotransmitters you generate in any given situation; your actions, attitudes and activities influence which tickets you purchase, which bus you can take and ultimately what experience you have. Persistent pain can be your body's way of alerting you that you have made a few wrong turns so that you take the correct bus the next time.

As in any major transport operation there needs to be a traffic controller to manage the flow, checking tickets, stopping traffic where needed and allowing buses through. In a tripartite synapse that traffic controller is an immune cell, known as an astrocyte, and these cells significantly influence the flow of neurotransmitters through the synaptic space and therefore the flow of information from the external world to your brain.[11] Generally once the controller has let one type of signal through, there isn't a need to let the same one through again if nothing else has changed externally. Unless the controller is extremely vigilant. This is where set points come in.

Each synapse has a set point or threshold at which the controller will allow neurotransmitters to cross the synaptic space. If that set point changes, the controller alters the flow of neurotransmitters allowed through, increasing or reducing the flow of messages through the system. This happens to a greater or lesser extent throughout your nervous system. Your body learns to recognise threatening tissue or cell activity, as well as dangerous or threatening behaviour and situations, and this will influence the threshold of the synapse.

Imagine that this huge transport system inside you has a surveillance network of CCTV cameras looking out for dangerous or suspicious behaviour. When it recognises something that it perceives as a threat, it will lower the set point. That increases the flow of messages through the synapse, including those from nociceptive fibres to potentially produce a pain experience. This means that if your body is under perceived threat, you are more likely to stimulate an existing pain pathway, or bus route, and have a flare-up of persistent pain.[12]

Your body is constantly learning and updating. Your immune system learns to protect you against infection by developing signalling systems to help it recognise microorganisms that are not associated with human cells. These unique microbial molecules are called pathogen-associated molecular patterns, or PAMPs. We have similarly unique molecular patterns for stressed, injured or infected human cells, such as in a musculoskeletal injury: these are referred to as danger-associated molecular patterns, or DAMPs. It's possible that we also have associated molecular patterns for behaviour, or BAMPs, such as encountering an angry dog or someone who acts threateningly towards you; cognitive-associated molecular patterns, or CAMPs, such as being bullied psychologically; and exogenous-associated molecular patterns, or XAMPs, such as foreign chemicals in the body like opioids.[13,14,15,16]

When you have a flu-like virus, you often get joint pain, a backache and sore muscles. This is because the virus's PAMP has lowered your synapse set point, making you more likely to experience pain. You haven't injured your back: instead you experience back pain because the set point has been altered in the presence of a virus. If you have a history of back pain (as most people do

26

at some stage in their life,[17] then you have an existing pathway for that pain. The set point being lowered can mean you set a bus or two off on that old pain pathway again even though you haven't hurt yourself.

In Chapter 1 I described pain as being like parking sensors in a car, designed to beep before you hit the wall. If the set point of the synapse is too low, your sensors will beep faster and louder. A stressful, pro-inflammatory life can make your controller overly vigilant, lowering the set point and leaving your pain system sensitised, heightening your signalling system to perceived danger. The pain that often ensues is not a reliable indicator of damage but an indicator that you are living a pro-inflammatory lifestyle and pain is perhaps the only way your body can alert you to this. It is a mentor, after all, there to help you consider such things. Unfortunately what often happens as a consequence of a pain flare-up is that you stop doing the things that are good for you because you fear that if you do, you will somehow harm yourself. This can reinforce that pain pathway, which makes it more likely to happen again. The problem gets compounded and keeps the set point low[18] unless you recalibrate it. We will look at how to recalibrate your set point later.

The pain is not imagined. It is very real. It happens because of signals being processed in the body. The difficulty is that these signals are not always processed in a way that means "hurt equals harm", as you might perceive. The pain system is trying to grab your attention but not because you've damaged something. It is trying to protect you. Pain is trying to tell you something – most likely that your life is more pro-inflammatory than you realised. Pain learns, it becomes swifter, it gets complicated and sometimes it gets in your way unless you know how to read it.

Brendan hurt his back doing some DIY. It was a simple mechanical back problem, and after a course of treatment with me he made a full recovery. He started going to the gym regularly, lifting some weights and even starting to run for the first time in his life. Brendan had recently retired and was enjoying this new level of fitness. All was well until he returned some months later with a flare-up of pain, which he blamed on picking up a towel from the floor. He thought he must have "bent down wrong", thereby damaging his back. This didn't make sense to me: he was lifting far heavier things in the gym with no problem. After some reassurance, a bit of stretching for a couple of days and a return to his usual training programme, all seemed well again. But this started to become a pattern. His back would be fine and then he'd have a sudden flare-up of pain. Each time he attributed the cause of the pain to bending and twisting, always for something innocuous such as picking up a small bag of shopping or tying his shoes.

We had several conversations, trying to figure out why his body was protecting him so vigorously. Eventually the answer came in the form of a case of wine. I was sure he must be under some sort of stress, which was stimulating his inflammatory system, priming his nociceptors to react to any potential threat. Brendan didn't agree with this, declaring he was not under stress. After a little more discussion, it turned out he was having some building work done which he found quite stressful, although he didn't want to admit that initially. He didn't like confrontation so didn't challenge the builders, but he was increasingly frustrated that they were making a mess. Each morning he went to the gym and generally felt good for doing so, but the rest of the day was spent either micromanaging the builders or tidying up after them and getting wound up about their messiness. He could feel the tension rising within him as the day went on, but he still couldn't see a link between this tension and his back pain.

During our conversations he mentioned that he enjoyed drinking wine and had a case delivered every few weeks. I asked him if his back ever "went" lifting the case of wine. He smiled and said never. Why was that? did he think. He smiled again and said, "Because I like wine." Wine didn't represent a threat.

We dissected the various manoeuvres involved in getting a case of wine from the front door of an apartment building, going up various flights of stairs, opening doors, bending up and down a dozen times to put each bottle in the wine fridge. Brendan started to reconsider his association of pain with lifting and twisting. He also started to question whether his recurring back pain was still a reliable indicator of harm or damage.

In the end his solution was to go to the gym in the late afternoon. By going in the morning, all his good work was being undone as he buried himself in the stress of the building job. Going to the gym in the afternoon got him away from the builders, reducing his exposure to stress and emptying his stress bucket, leaving him more relaxed and less tense. Brendan enjoyed his evening more. He slept better, he started his days feeling less irritable and with some capacity to deal with the challenges of the building work. He trusted that he was OK to lift and twist. In fact, it was good for him. Needless to say, his back pain didn't resurface.

To sum up, the first part of the pain pathway is sensory data: information that comes from the outside world via the senses to the spinal cord. Nociceptive fibres help distinguish between safe and potentially dangerous stimuli. These fibres are sensitised by inflammation, so a stressful, pro-inflammatory lifestyle will make you more likely to experience pain and will contribute to flare-ups. Your body sends signals up the spinal cord to the brain for interpretation if a particular threshold, or set point, is reached. How that threshold is regulated is influenced by potential threats such as infection, tissue trauma, pro-inflammatory lifestyles, threatening behaviour or cognitive stress. What is considered safe or potentially dangerous will be different for everyone.

In Chapters 11 and 12, we'll be looking at the parts of the brain involved in storing and retaining data, and how your brain uses those data to filter information from the sensory part of the pathway to help you navigate through life. This is a complex process, sometimes leading to misunderstandings about what is causing persistent pain and why. We'll explore how such misunderstandings can have a radical effect on how you experience the world and interpret persistent pain, as well as how to recalibrate a sensitised pain pathway to work in your favour. Before that, it's time to think about your own health hexagon – which contributes to generating such data in the first place.

CHAPTER 4

How to Think About Balance

AS I SET OUT in the introduction, this book focuses on the six aspects of life that are essential to your overall well-being. These six elements make up what I call your health hexagon, and we will shortly be looking at each one in turn. First, though, I want to talk about balance.

At different stages of life, the amount of time you need to allocate to each part of your hexagon will vary depending on the demands on you and your goals. If you are trying to establish a career or build a business, you will spend more time in that mental/cognitive space. If you have children, there will be a greater demand in the emotional space. If you retire, or your children leave home, or you get sick, or the things you do to relax are unavailable, you will need to recalibrate. Life will constantly throw up uncertainty, and you must have some capacity to deal with these known unknowns. Here are three key principles I have found particularly useful in thinking about balance.

No such thing as average

In *Rebel Ideas*, Matthew Syed tells the story of the US Air Force in the late 1940s and early 1950s, a period when they were struggling with a high volume of accidents.[1] In February 1950 alone the Air Force recorded 172 incidents – not all fatalities but a large volume of near misses – and they needed a solution. After much investigation Lieutenant Gilbert S. Daniels, a Harvard graduate who specialised in physical anthropology, concluded that the cockpit design must be the issue, having ruled out pilot training, engineering and electrical faults. The cockpit was designed for the average pilot. Pilots were preselected to meet specific height criteria, so the range of possible heights was already narrow. Daniels selected 4,063 pilots and measured 140 variables on each subject, including their height, weight, waist size, femur length, thumb length and so on.

When the analysis was complete and the numbers crunched, he looked to see how many pilots fell into the "average" category. The surprising answer was that out of 4,063 pilots, not one pilot was average. In seeking to make the cockpit suitable for everyone, they had made it suitable for no one. The solution was to make the cockpit seat and joystick adjustable. The result? The number of accidents plummeted.

We see this time and time again when trying to aim for some recommended average or ideal. Health industries love a template to work from. Systems are built around averages and bell curves. Advice on how to live is often based on following or attaining the typical or average for any series of metrics. This can be a reasonable starting point when thinking about a population. The body mass index, or BMI, uses two variables, height and weight, to formulate a scale of healthy or unhealthy weight. It is then used to help predict the risk of illness such as heart disease, diabetes and osteoarthritis. You can't change your height of course, unless you are still growing (or shrinking in latter years), but you can change your weight, and doing so will change where you are on the BMI spectrum, perhaps moving you from "unhealthy" to "healthy".

The difficulty with BMI is that it is flawed for an individual. Take a professional rugby player whose weight consists of lean muscle mass and another individual of similar height whose weight consists of excessive fat storage. Both could be high on a BMI scale and deemed unhealthy, but their situations are completely different. I'm not saying that BMI doesn't have its place – but you are an individual, not an average, and you need to consider any data or recommendation within your personal context and circumstances.

The 50:40:10 rule

Professor Sonja Lyubomirsky's 50:40:10 rule has been widely applied to different contexts. Here I'm using it as a guide to navigating your risk of illness or injury and therefore health and well-being. Broadly speaking, 50 per cent of such risk is determined by your genes. This includes your anatomy. If everyone in your family as far back as you can remember has had a heart attack or needed a knee replacement, there is a fifty-fifty chance you'll suffer the same fate.

Forty per cent of your risk is determined by lifestyle. How you live has a big influence on your health and well-being. If you are a professional footballer, a marathon runner or overweight, you are going to wear your knees out quicker than most, and if you also have that strong family history of knee replacements, you may be 90 per cent of the way to needing a replacement yourself. If you have a strong family history of heart disease and eat unhealthily, smoke and drink excessively, don't exercise and have a stressful life, you're a heart attack waiting to happen.

Ten per cent will be determined by comorbidities and circumstances. This does not mean some form of entirely random

33

bad luck but rather accidents, previous injuries or other illnesses. Think of the footballer with a strong family history of knee arthritis who suffers a bad tackle and tears some cartilage or ligaments. That will make the need for a knee replacement in their lifetime highly likely. For someone with a heart condition, such 10-per cent factors might include an infection causing damage to the heart or perhaps side effects of medications for other conditions being treated. There is a link between gum disease and heart disease, for example, so looking after your teeth properly could also fall into that 10 per cent. Where you live will also be part of your circumstances – air quality, exposure to daylight, how much space you have. Let's say you are very tall but are living and working in a world designed for the "average" person, cramming yourself into a small desk and chair. This will have an impact on how your body performs and what you expose it to.

We can't really change our genes – well, not yet anyway – so that makes the other two elements all the more important. You have a certain amount of control over your own lifestyle and circumstances – both of which may even influence the way your genes behave. If you have a strong family history of knee replacements, for example, you might consider cycling rather than running, avoid contact sports and focus on maintaining a healthy weight. That might just prevent you from needing a knee replacement. Register the hand that life has dealt you as this will have an impact on how your life choices influence your health.

Bucket theory

You've probably come across the simple concept of the bucket theory. If you keep filling a bucket with water, eventually it will overflow. Now apply the analogy to yourself: if you take on too much, you will eventually get beyond your capacity and life will become challenging and stressful, perhaps painful. You need to do something to bail water out of the bucket. That might be a good night's sleep, which gives you some capacity again. Your pain reduces or disappears, you feel less anxious, you have space to think.

It's easy to assume that the bucket analogy is a 24-hour cycle, and you start off with an empty bucket every day. Sadly this is not the case. Everything you do will have an impact on using up some capacity, and your ability to bail out the water will depend on your lifestyle too. On any given day your capacity can vary – some days a 5 km run is no problem and on others it puts you over the top. It's easy to assume you've done something wrong on those occasions, but it's more likely that you simply didn't have enough capacity. Perhaps your bucket was already 90 per cent full before you started and therefore it doesn't take much to overflow. It's not the activity; it's doing it on top of everything else that's going on.

How much physical activity you do isn't just the number of miles you run or cycle or swim. It's everything you are doing at a physical level. I see patients all the time who say they haven't over-done it because they run for only 30 minutes three times a week. This isn't a huge amount for many people, but it's all about the wider context. What if you also work on your feet all day? What if you have a large garden and you mow it by hand a couple of times a week and you play football with the kids or grandchildren every weekend? What if your hobby is building boats and you also love a bit of DIY each week? What if you always stay up late and get up early every morning? What if some weeks you miss a couple of runs and end up doing one run for 90 minutes? What if your partner is sick and you're worried they are going to lose their job?

The bucket fills up with physical, emotional and environmental stresses, and life is a balancing act of emptying the bucket quicker than you fill it up. If you overflow regularly, then you need to make some changes to your lifestyle to live within your capacity. You can also improve your overall capacity – that is, get a bigger bucket – by improving your tolerance for certain stresses. An exercise training programme can improve your fitness, strength and resilience to physical loads. Understanding yourself better can aid your mental capacity. Learning to relax effectively can help keep your bucket from overflowing in the first place. This is what the health hexagon is all about, figuring out what you need in each part of your life. Perhaps when your cognitive stress bucket is full, spending time in the physical space can help bail out your mental stress bucket: filling one empties another. It's a little like the law of the conservation of energy, which says that energy cannot be created or destroyed, but rather transferred from one form to another.[2]

It isn't always easy to understand which bucket you are filling up at any given time, though, and usually you'll be filling and emptying more than one at any point anyway. Which ones are ready to spill over and which ones have plenty of space is a constant calculation. How much capacity you have for any given area of your life will depend on many factors – as described in the 50:40:10 principle – but the size of the bucket you need and the one you have can be different.

Let's take exercise as an example. You like the idea of running but you are not a runner. You fantasise about it, dreaming that not only could you run a marathon but you might even win the thing. Surely it's just walking fast, and you've being doing that for years. Yet a quick dash up the stairs is enough to leave you out of breath, with aching thighs and a stiff hip. Your running bucket is going to

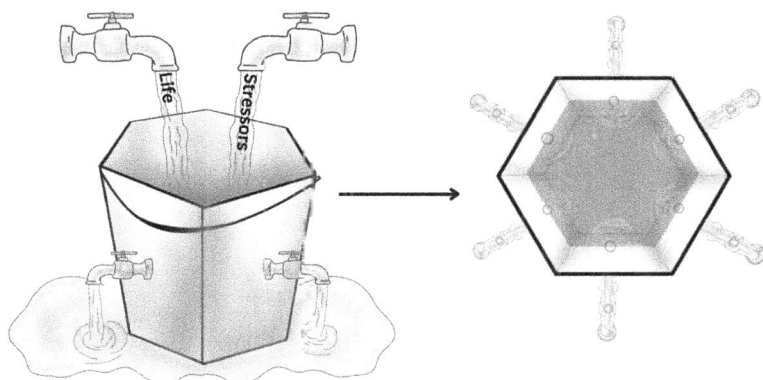

Figure 2: The Bucket Theory

Life and its stressors are like taps filling a bucket (your capacity). The six elements of the health hexagon (Mental, Physical, Spiritual, Emotional, Sleep and Diet) are outlet valves to create space for the continuous demands and challenges that life involves. If you don't have a reliable system (health hexagon) to empty the bucket quicker than it fills up, you will overflow, often resulting in a persistent pain flare-up.

need some serious capacity, and you've got something resembling a teacup. How do you turn that teacup into a reservoir? You train, slowly but surely. The amazing thing about the body is that it is organic and capable of change and development.

Now there's a question that's bound to come up during that training process. Why is it that sometimes you do something and it doesn't hurt, and then you do the same thing again and it really hurts? Have you injured yourself? Are you getting worse rather than better?

In very simple terms, stuff hurts because of capacity. Every structure in the body, whether a ligament, tendon, muscle, bone or joint, has a certain capacity to tolerate load. In most cases load is good: for example, you need to do weight-bearing exercise to maintain or improve your bone density to prevent osteoporosis. Astronauts need to spend time on a treadmill to give their bones some shock to prevent bone loss while in space. Tendons like load as it keeps them strong. Muscles respond to load and get bigger. But every structure has a threshold at which there is a maximum load it can accept. Beyond that, it will start to experience stress; in response it will stimulate some pain or discomfort. Some stress stimulates the tissue to adapt and get stronger, but if the load is too great that structure will fail, resulting in, say, a ruptured tendon or broken bone.

If you break a bone, its capacity to tolerate load will be minimal, but part of the healing process will be to get that bone to accept more load to stimulate its repair. Over time you will progress from non-weight-bearing on two crutches to partial weight-bearing at 25 per cent, 50 per cent, 75 per cent and eventually to fully weight-bearing. Then you will need to steadily build up that ability for longer periods until you can increase the load further by running, jumping and so on. This process has to be done gradually and in line with your individual capability. Going from completely non-weight-bearing to jumping won't work and will create bigger problems. The aim is to put the right amount of stress on tissues to get them to adapt. This is true whether you are recovering from injury or training to get fitter. When you exercise, you generate micro-trauma, breaking down the structures ever so slightly to kick-start a healing response. If the rate of repair is greater than the rate of breakdown, you get stronger.

At this point I must point out that hurt doesn't necessarily equal harm. It's OK for things to hurt sometimes; understanding why is the key. When you start weight-bearing on a recovering fracture, it's likely to be uncomfortable. Doing it under the guidance of an experienced clinician will help you safely navigate the discomfort as you build your strength.

Knowing where that line is between discomfort and development is a juggling act. In some cases, you will need expert guidance and in others, you can figure it out as you go. Decades of research have gone into a host of training programs to establish the right amount of stress to put the body under (and the necessary periods of recovery) in order to achieve certain goals. The mistake that most people make is to see this training programme in isolation. They perceive that the only time they are putting stuff into their bucket is when they are out running or lifting weights. In reality, you are filling up and emptying out all the time.

Figuring out this process isn't just about exercise either – it applies to all aspects of life. Have you ever noticed how, when you're feeling good, minor irritations seem to bother you less, whereas on days when you're feeling stressed, something as trivial as a botched coffee order or an uncomfortable chair can push you over the edge? The real problem is generally not the offending chair or wrong drink; it's your capacity to cope.

So, what does all this mean for you? It's easy to read an article or watch a documentary and think that veganism or the 5:2 diet is the answer; that Pilates or transcendental meditation or a sit-stand desk will fix everything. Unfortunately it is rarely that simple, and there is no one-size-fits-all solution. If there is anything we know, it's that no two people have the same life experiences and no one is truly average. You are flying your own plane, so you must set it up to work best for you.

What is it that fills your bucket and what helps empty it? Try not to think of any one activity being good or bad but rather as drops into the bucket: as long as you're taking enough out, you'll be able to put more in. It's worth considering that the degree to which something fills or empties the bucket will also vary from person to person. A good night's sleep is universally restorative but might bail out 50 per cent for your bucket and only 10 per cent for someone else's. Can you analyse what works for you? Just don't have too many variables in play at any one time while you're doing it. Sometimes the same thing can both fill and empty your bucket. Some forms of exercise may empty more than they fill, whereas more exercise isn't necessarily better.

All this talk of buckets is well and good, but what does it have to do with pain? you might ask. When your bucket is full you are exceeding your capacity and therefore heading for a pro-inflammatory lifestyle. We know this sensitises your nociceptive fibres, but it also lowers the set point of the astrocytes, heightening the central nervous system's vigilance and resulting in nociplastic pain. Pain is the mentor that lets you know your bucket is full and that it's time to check in with your health hexagon.

One last consideration when it comes to balance. If you get diagnosed with a disease, chances are you will want to learn about the condition. You may end up knowing a great deal about it, but that expertise is likely to pale in comparison to the consultant who's been working in that field for years. Equally the consultant has some knowledge of what you're going through from their experience of seeing thousands of patients over the years, but they don't know what it feels like to be a patient unless they too have been one, and even then they still can't know what it feels like to be you. When you seek the help of an expert, remember there are two experts in the room: them – and you. It will be up to you to figure out what part of their advice is suitable for you. Don't accept it or dismiss it entirely just because it doesn't fit into your current thinking. I hope this book can in some part help you make an informed decision.

Let's explore the hexagon and how the actions, activities and attitudes you adopt in each branch can make for a pro- or anti-inflammatory lifestyle.

CHAPTER 5

The Physical Space

BEING ACTIVE IS about much more than sport. It includes moving regularly, doing the housework, gardening, taking the stairs instead of the lift, walking instead of driving, getting that thing yourself rather than asking the kids to do it. Simple stuff, but it all adds up.

I don't want to give you a formula for exercise but rather a framework through which you can figure out what is enough for you. In this chapter we'll look at how exercise affects the neurotransmitters that help regulate your stress and pain system; some of the common misconceptions around exercise; how to choose the correct exercise for you; fatigue and flexibility; how to measure performance; and how to set yourself up for success when it comes to physical activity.

Some biochemistry

Endorphins and endocannabinoids are sometimes described as the body's natural painkillers. They get released when you exert yourself physically and contribute to the euphoria you might notice after exercise.[1] Physical effort doesn't have to just be traditional exercise like running, jumping or swimming – a good day's labour can give you the same 'buzz". Over time, as you get fitter, you have to push yourself harder to get that same buzz from exercise.

As you stress your body physically, you will also release stress hormones such as norepinephrine and adrenaline, which will help with things like glucose release for energy and increasing your heart rate to get that glucose to various muscles to burn.

In moderation, physical stress can strengthen your body, reducing your risk of injury and illness.[2] But too much stress, physical or otherwise, can threaten your immune system and leave you vulnerable to infection, lower your set points, heighten your pain sensitivity and fill your bucket more than it empties. As always, it's about balance: figuring out what is enough for you and what is sustainable within the context of your health hexagon.

Exercise has also been linked to the release of dopamine, the neurotransmitter of reward or success.[3] When you score a goal or progress towards a milestone, you get a hit of dopamine. You get the same sense of achievement from other physical activities, such as gardening or fixing that leaking tap. Whatever it is though, you need to pay attention: if you don't realise you've scored the goal, you don't get the dopamine hit. We'll come back to selective attention when we look at pain more closely in Chapter 11.

If you watch golf on TV, you can get a skewed opinion of what is normal. Golf coverage tends to focus on the successes, rarely showing you the short putts missed by these experts in their field. This can make you think that you as a golfer should be knocking putts in from at least 10 and 12 feet away all the time. If you look at the statistics of professional tour golfers, their success rate of sinking a putt from 8 feet is remarkably only 50 per cent. Half the time these elite performers are missing putts the length of a dining room table. If you expect to make every putt from 12, 15 or 20 feet, you are going to be disappointed. If you get one from 10 feet but believe there is nothing special about that, then you won't get the dopamine hit you should have. You've had a win but haven't realised it because you're being too hard on yourself.

Exercise has been shown to raise serotonin levels, which lift our mood and boost our confidence. This neurotransmitter has also been linked to appetite regulation and sleep quality. Serotonin is also influenced by your sense of where you are in a particular hierarchy. If you perceive yourself to be higher up that hierarchy, you will have a greater sense of self-confidence and higher serotonin levels. If you are higher up the league tables in your local tennis club, fit for your age for your run, swim or cycle, have a lower handicap in golf, score a higher break in snooker or get closer to the target in archery than the person beside you, it's likely to influence your serotonin levels. Be wary of unhelpful comparisons though: if you're always comparing yourself to people you perceive as better than you, you may end up with a more distorted view of yourself at the bottom of any hierarchy, which is not going to help your confidence.

Remember, these neurotransmitters are the tickets you purchase for the various buses you take within your sensory system. I've given only a brief example of a few neurotransmitters that exercise can influence: you will need to figure out how much exercise and what type works best for you and when to compete or not. You have significant control over what these neurotransmitters are by the hexagon lifestyle you engineer.

Who are you comparing yourself to?

Many patients tell me how demoralising it is that everyone in their yoga class is so much better than they are. Often the problem is that they are looking at it the wrong way. People are generally under the impression that muscles are elastic bands and that they stretch. This is not the case. Muscles are more like chains and the links in the chain slide over and back on each other. This is how a muscle gets longer or shorter. How many links you have in the chain comes down to genes, not how often you exercise.

Yoga classes tend to attract people who are naturally flexible. Genetically they are likely to have more links in their chains than your average person. I won't go into the details of connective tissue and hypermobility conditions and the difference between flexibility and elasticity and collagen make-up and distribution; the point is, if these people never did a stretch again for the rest of their lives, they'd still be able to touch their toes.

People who are flexible may gravitate towards yoga because they are good at it – and being good at something makes them feel good. They may not be fully aware that this is why they enjoy it, and, in many ways, it doesn't matter. It works for them, so that's great. But they are not necessarily the people who will benefit most from a yoga class.

If a muscle is held in a shortened position for long periods of time, like sitting down at a desk all day, then the body can lose links in the chain. Your body is replenishing tissue all the time: if you don't use it, the body will put that protein elsewhere. That's why muscles can shorten and feel tight. With regular stretching, you can stimulate the body to grow more links in the chain but only back to your predetermined genetic threshold. Someone with tight hamstrings who struggles to bend forward but gets a little bit better with each session will benefit their muscles far more at a structural level than the person whose head can reach between their knees.

The progress is what counts. That's what gives you the dopamine. So don't compare yourself to the super-flexible person beside you. You are going somewhere. Recognise that and you will get the serotonin, dopamine and endorphins that help reduce pain and stress. If you feel like a failure because of how you're looking at the situation, you'll get the opposite. Work out what game you are in. Try to understand what you are aiming for. Recognise where you are making progress so you can see some achievement and get the neurotransmitters you deserve.

So is the super flexible person doing yoga wasting their time? Not at all. Exercise isn't about just the mechanics of the exercise, but so much more. There is the community, the identity, the feeling that you are good at something, the discipline of going, the switching off from the outside world, the relaxation, the breathing, the stress relief, a sense of being connected to something bigger than yourself. It is worth thinking about what exactly it's doing for you though – over time that flexible person might find it more beneficial to focus on improving a different element of their physical fitness. Working on their bone density or speed or power may improve their hexagon more. Maybe you are the big strong guy in the gym lifting the biggest weights, but you've got loads of back pain or had multiple hernia operations. Is it really working for you? It could be time to mix things up a bit.

Is all exercise good exercise?

I get asked a lot if one specific exercise is better than another. That all depends on what you are trying to achieve with that exercise and how it fits with your health hexagon. Exercise works at many levels. Although we are focusing on the physical in this chapter, rarely is any one activity exclusive to a single arm of the hexagon. If you are part of an exercise group, for example, it's as much about the group spirit and the emotional space as it is about the actual exercise you are doing.

Rather than thinking about good or bad exercise, the more helpful question is what exercise are you doing and what do you need it for? If you need weight-bearing exercise for your bone health, things like walking and running will be better than non-weight-bearing exercise, such as swimming or cycling. If you sit down all day for your job, then it's probably best not to sit on a bike or rowing machine when you exercise. Your body needs variety of movement. But what if you sit at a desk *and* you're passionate about cycling? Well – you can still make space in your hexagon for cycling of course, but you may want to stretch a bit more or do some walking or running to complement it. Chances are if you are getting the balance wrong, your body will let you know by making something stiff and sore. This doesn't mean it's damaged; it may just be letting you know you need to improve other areas. That's what pain does. It tries to protect you, grab your attention and nudge you to change something.

Next: where are you exercising? Thinking about your hexagon in broad terms, I would suggest getting outside. This way you get some fresh air and exposure to daylight, which will help your vitamin D levels and calibrate your circadian rhythm to help your sleep cycle. You can change your pace and direction more easily and more often, which will improve your balance, and you will be exposed to a variety of stimuli. You might even bump into someone you know, which will give you a little hit of oxytocin, a neurotransmitter that helps with bonding, security and emotional well-being.

If you just look at the exercise in a mechanical sense (i.e. running is running regardless of where you do it), you are missing the point of how exercise fits into your health hexagon for your overall wellness. Maybe the treadmill in the gym works well for you because you love getting to watch football on the TV at the same time. If so, great. My point is, there are other factors to consider in determining which type of exercise brings you the greatest benefit.

Of course, you may see many obstacles to exercising. I challenge you to examine whether these are genuine blocks or surmountable challenges:

- *I don't have the time.* Is every minute of your day really used efficiently? You'll probably find that if you exercise consistently, it will help you get more organised and free up some time.
- *The weather is bad.* You only need the right clothes to overcome this obstacle. Everyone's ideal weather is different anyway – someone somewhere in the world would be delighted for it to be colder and wetter or dryer and hotter than how it is for you right now.
- *It's not nice where I live.* If you don't like your surroundings, take an audiobook with you or go somewhere else to exercise. It's never going to be perfect, but you are a grown-up, so take some responsibility for yourself.
- *I have to pick the kids up from school.* Great, how about you walk there and walk them home? That way they get a walk too. Your kids will pay more attention to what you do than what you say, and walking or running to pick them up from school sets a culture for your family that will stay with them forever.

It's easy to obsess about certain exercises being good or bad or right or wrong. It's also easy to get fixated on technique and worry that you are going to damage yourself if you do it ever so slightly wrong. Neither mindset is going to help you. The fear of doing things wrong can get in the way of doing anything at all. You are not as fragile as you think. The margin of error on technique is often greater than you realise, so if you are not doing things perfectly, don't panic. The anxiety of "getting it wrong" can be more problematic than the technique itself.

The purpose of exercise is to improve, achieve manageable goals so that you can set new goals and feel good. Doing something is usually better than doing nothing – the evidence suggests that almost any exercise is good for persistent non-specific low back pain.[4] The questions to ask yourself when it comes to physical activity are: Are you making progress? Are you gaining confidence in your body by doing it? Does it help move you closer to whatever it is you are aiming for? Maybe you want a faster time or a chance to escape. Whatever it is, keep checking in to decide what is enough, whether it's working for you or whether there's a better way. Get some help and advice along the way to guide you, but be careful where you get that expertise from. Your stored data will retain the advice and experiences you have: for example, if you're fixated on keeping your back straight on a particular exercise, is that really necessary?

Boom and bust

When it comes to exercise it's also important to be fit for your sport, not fit by your sport. By this I mean that there is more to being able to do an exercise than just the exercise itself. In clinic I regularly see people with injuries because they don't condition their bodies for their sport. Professional swimmers spend a lot more time working on their fitness outside of the pool than you might imagine. Working the appropriate muscles in the gym to prevent injury and maximise performance in the pool can be essential. Depending on your chosen sport and your own strengths and weaknesses, you will need to consider which areas need a little more attention to help you get fit for your sport. There is no one-size-fits-all fix.

Having some reliability and consistency to your exercise routine helps, as does making sure you can sustain that routine and minimise the risk of being derailed by injury. A balanced exercise programme will be useful here. You may not enjoy doing a stretching routine or core exercises as you don't have enough time and all you want to do is get out on the tennis court and play, but how would you feel if you then found you couldn't play for 6 to 12 weeks because you had picked up some overload injury? How would that affect your neurotransmitters and your astrocytes?

Playing tennis three times a week and a couple of core sessions on the non-playing days might prove to be the sustainable formula for you rather than five days of tennis a week for a bit and then dropping out. Perhaps you've noticed a pattern. You play five days a week for a few months but then you are injured again and out for a few more. It's super frustrating and puts your hexagon out of balance in the meantime because you might be a nightmare to live or work with if you are not getting your tennis fix.

Think of exercise like making a cake. The ingredients are the specific exercises themselves: stretching, aerobics, resistance, endurance. You need to mix them together in the right quantities to get the cake you want. That mix must go in the oven for the correct amount of time (the frequency and duration of time you devote to exercise in your week). The oven needs to be at the right temperature (the intensity of your exercise). Depending on your cake mix, you might be aiming for a sponge, a souffle or a pancake. If you cook it at too high a temperature or for too long, it'll get burnt. Too low or too short a time and that mix is staying sloppy. Exercise is a form of alchemy, an art as well as a science, and you need to experiment to get the variables just right. When you don't, your pain mentor will let you know.

Consider the ingredients you have to work with in the first place and what you are hoping to achieve. No amount of bodybuilding will turn Olympic champion Mo Farah into a heavyweight boxer. I've seen patients over the years trying to train towards something they are not genetically designed for, and it rarely works out well. This isn't to say that being on that journey isn't beneficial. The destination isn't necessarily as important as the incremental improvements along the way. If you are starting an exercise plan with the belief that changing your body into something it was not designed to become will somehow fix all your troubles, you will be doubly disappointed. You have to play the hand you are dealt the best way you can. Trying to force unrealistic change can lead to destructive behaviour or practices such as taking steroids for bodybuilding. This will make things a whole lot worse, not better.

If you have persistent pain, the idea of playing tennis even once a week might seem impossible. That's OK, your journey is your own. Whatever level you are at physically, can you nudge it forward as you figure out what is enough for you? That might be walking for five minutes rather than running a marathon. Over time, five minutes can become longer and your options can expand. But there will be an optimum point somewhere after which you're looking at diminishing returns. More isn't necessarily better. You might discover that as other parts of your hexagon get more organised, your capacity in the physical space improves and you can do more with fewer pain flare-ups or boom-bust cycles. Or you might find that, as other areas of your hexagon improve, you actually need the gym less and are better off for it.

Timing is an important factor in exercise. You might need a little bit of time to get going in the morning before you ask your body too many questions. Some people can jump out of bed and get straight to an intense workout. Others perform much better in the afternoon or evening. Pay attention to what works best for you. If you have lots of other commitments there might not be a perfect time – but fitting it in at a less ideal time is better than not at all.

At one stage in my career, I did some work for a large pharmaceutical company. I used to arrive at 7.30 a.m. at my office, which was next to the gym with big shiny windows. At that hour of the morning, I would see the senior executives on the treadmills and bikes and rowing machines. At lunchtime I saw the professional staff such as the scientists and administrators attending different gym classes. At the end of the day, when most people had gone home, the gym was exclusively attended by the gym junkies. Everyone was using the gym for different reasons. The thing that struck me then was how on earth the senior executives had time for the gym. They were super busy people, flying around the world, with large departments to manage and every second of their day accounted for. What I now realise is that they were using the gym to manage their stress and help them prepare for the day ahead, and their appointment with the gym was just as important as any other one on their schedule.

Going back to the bucket theory of the previous chapter, it's worth asking yourself what your capacity for physical activity is on any given day and whether you are spreading that activity out at an appropriate rate. Patients frequently tell me that they run 10 miles or cycle 50 miles on a Sunday, but for the rest of the week they just sit at their desk. They then wonder why they are sore. Instead they might be better off running 3 to 5 miles three times a week. This way they would empty their bucket more frequently and the regular training would allow better tissue adaptation and give them a bigger bucket in the long run so that eventually a 10-mile run at the weekend wouldn't exceed their capacity.

So, is all exercise good exercise? Are some exercises better than others? Everyone has their own answer to these questions – it depends on you, your lifestyle and what you need exercise to achieve for you.

Understand who you are

Your personality will have a big impact on what you need from exercise. If you're a highly conscientious person, you're likely to feel obligated to stick to your exercise plan. This can be positive, helping you to succeed where others drop away. It can also work against you if plans and priorities change as life gets in the way. Your exercise routine needs to be robust but also flexible enough that it can adapt to change. If you typically run three times a week on specific days, it's no big deal if you need to change days or miss an occasional run. It all balances out in the end, and that flexibility allows you to keep the bigger picture in mind. There are other people in your life whose needs will sometimes conflict with yours; sometimes your attention is required elsewhere. That's life – and being able to adapt will help you keep your hexagon balanced overall.

People who score lower on conscientiousness might need more support and encouragement from others to help them succeed. Understanding your personality type will allow you to put systems in place to help manage your natural tendency to avoid exercise, such as buddying up with a friend for walks or runs, joining a class or getting a personal trainer. To succeed you need to know where you want to be heading to (i.e. you want to be more physically active). You have to acknowledge where you are now (that you are less fit than you should be). And you also have to take the necessary action to get to your destination, such as joining a class and going to every session. If you genuinely want to change you will put these processes in place, but most importantly, you need a reason to do the things you instinctively don't like doing (For more on this, see the 12-point plan at the end of this chapter.)

Some people find it easy to allow exercise to become a crutch. I have seen many patients whose relationship with exercise has been destructive and unhealthy, but because exercise is often viewed as a good thing, it can be harder to identify in yourself and others that it is a problem. Exercise is generally helpful, but the dose needs to be optimum. Having to exercise more and more to "feel normal" may indicate that there is an issue.

The CAGE questionnaire is often used as a tool to see if someone has a substance abuse problem, but it can be a good starting point to think about how healthy your relationship with exercise is. Answering yes to two or more of these questions could indicate a problem and might alert you to the need for some professional help. The questions are as follows:

1. Have you felt the need to **C**ut down on your exercise?
2. Have people **A**nnoyed you by criticising your relationship with exercise?

3. Have you felt **G**uilty about your exercise?
4. Is it the first thing you think about in the morning, or have you felt the need to exercise in the morning to feel normal – an **E**ye-opener?

If you are naturally competitive and tend to obsess over succeeding or setting yourself even bigger challenges, be careful what you start. Can you set some rules for yourself so that the amount of exercise you do works for your hexagon overall? Do you have enough space in your life for another goal or challenge right now? Would that be fair on the people you live with and would the training or event clash with pinch points in your work? Maybe what is right for you is running 5 km regularly but not opening the door to half marathons and marathons because you want to keep the other parts of your hexagon balanced.

Remember who you are and what you are exercising for. I see numerous patients who are trying to train like a professional athlete while also working a full-time job. If you are a professional sportsperson, then the physical space of your hexagon will be more cognitive. You're likely to be focusing on sports science, technique, nutrition and recovery strategies in far greater detail than any amateur needs to. Professional athletes rest much more than most of us realise. They often have a nap in the day after a training session to help with recovery as well as a minimum of eight to nine hours' sleep a night. If you are trying to copy the training schedule of an Olympian while also juggling work, family and everything else going on in your life, then you are going to struggle. That's not to say you can't learn from the professionals, but think carefully about how much capacity you have to spare. Your mentor will make you aware if necessary.

Ride the wave

New Zealand-born Dave "Rasta" Rastovich was a world-class surfer on the professional tour with the brightest of futures ahead of him. A sponsor's dream, he had the admiration of his colleagues and an ability to ride any wave anywhere. And then, seemingly out of nowhere he quit the sport aged just 20.

To people inside and outside the surfing world, this was madness. He was at the top of his game, with all the endorsements and trappings of success that go with it. What's not to love? But that was the point. He'd fallen out of love with it.

As a kid growing up along the sunshine coast of Australia, Rasta fell in love with surfing. The ocean was where he felt alive, where he felt at peace and where he felt he needed to be. Surfing was as fundamental and as vital as breathing. It seemed only natural that he would end up making his living from it too.

Driving home from an event where he finished runner-up, however, that all changed. He'd been beaten. It happens – no one wins all the time, right? That's what he couldn't get his head around. He was out on the waves that day having an amazing time. Absolutely in the moment, in the zone, where he was always meant to be. And then came the scores.

Someone else decided that he wasn't having as good a time as he thought he was. Someone else decided that today he wasn't good enough. That just didn't make sense to him. Why was he letting his enjoyment of surfing be measured by someone else? He loved what he did today, but that feeling was destroyed by a score placed on his experience. As a consequence, he felt miserable for the rest of the day. He had failed. His sense of self had been threatened and his body biochemistry responded accordingly. All because of a score, a measure given by someone else's definition of success. And that's why he quit the tour.

Now, some might argue that he gave up. Maybe so, but that was his decision to make. He still surfs, and loves it as much as ever in fact. Maybe he's even better than ever, but no one else needs to know. No one's keeping score and he hasn't had a bad day on the waves since.[5] That's a pretty good result in my book.

We need to consider the same. Is this something you need to measure? Will a score motivate you and help you improve or make you feel anxious or like a failure? Are you measuring yourself against someone else's achievements – and is that the right comparator for you? If you're an athlete and working towards a particular goal – all well and good. If a target helps you get where you need to be and it's rebalancing your hexagon – go for it. But if it's taking more away from you than it's giving back, then it may be time to ditch the clock, the score, the scales. Have your run. Enjoy your run. Get it done and measure how you feel afterwards.

I've seen plenty of high achievers over the years who fixate on pushing themselves in every aspect of their lives. They end up seeing me because they are in persistent pain, so something about their hexagon isn't balanced. It can take a bit of work to help them understand that by measuring everything they do, they are adding pressure to an already full and stressful life.

You will need to decide which space exercise best fits into for you. If you are a professional athlete, exercise will unavoidably be more in the mental/cognitive space – for others, that's not necessary. If exercise is part of your overall wellness, do you need to measure everything about it? Maybe focus on how often you run rather than how quickly or slowly you move. Measure something else, something more important.

Fatigue

It's hard to exercise and you will feel fatigued as you do it or afterwards. Fatigue can also be caused by a number of medical conditions (including anaemia, diabetes and sleep apnoea, to name a few). Poor sleep quality in general and dehydration also contribute to fatigue. But these are not the only reasons we can feel fatigued.

The scientist Tim Noakes has spent his career looking at how the mind affects our sense of fatigue. He and others suggest that the brain works as a central governor, limiting our ability to push beyond perceived fatigue to ensure self-preservation. This was useful for hunter-gatherers who needed enough energy to get safely back to base before becoming so fatigued physically from the hunt that they became the hunted.

Noakes has shown that we will nearly always psychologically fatigue before we physiologically fatigue. In other words, our brains tell us to stop before our bodies need to.[6] If you've ever trained to improve your fitness such as doing Couch to 5K or pushed yourself on a big cycle or half marathon, you'll know there are many moments where you want to stop but you somehow find a way to keep going.

Wherever we set the finish line is where we fatigue. When we go out for a run, we subconsciously pace ourselves. So, if you are doing a 5 km run you will feel that the last 500 m or so are really hard work, but if you go out for an 8 km run or a 10 km run you won't feel the same level of fatigue until you get nearer that new finish line you've set yourself.

In life we set various finish lines all the time. Christmas is a perfect example. We look towards that date as a marker or finish line. We pace ourselves subconsciously to get to Christmas. Finish that piece of work and clear the decks before the end of the year and then as it approaches, we can feel fatigued, flat, fed up and worn out.

Of course, such finish lines are arbitrary and likely to move around. In life, nobody knows where the real finish line is. Pace yourself in your physical space. The goal is to have enough physical activity in your life for your whole life.

Exercise as medicine

Exercise has been shown to help in the prevention and management of 26 chronic diseases,[7] so it is an essential part of your health hexagon. Sedentary lifestyles mean you have to take responsibility for putting a system in place to make your exercise habitual. If you can do that, you'll have taken care of one-sixth of your lifestyle and you don't have to think about it much more beyond that.

If you're in persistent pain, all this talk about running and marathons might sound so unapplicable that you dismiss this chapter as irrelevant. Exercise is medicine and progress is the therapy. So even if that's a few steps, a few push-ups or a stretch, it's heading in the right direction and improving your capacity, your health hexagon, to alter your astrocytes, your set points, your stored data and your pain experience.

I like to think I treat every patient I see in clinic as a professional athlete. They are just in a different race or game to those we see on the podium.

Exercise and how to keep doing it: the 12-point plan

The reality is that very few people enjoy exercising, but nearly everyone enjoys the benefits of exercise. In 25 years of being a physiotherapist working with clients ranging from grassroots players to Olympic contenders, I can assure you that very few people indeed enjoy exercise. Even the world champions. People like games but, by and large, what they enjoy is less doing the actual exercise and more the feeling of well-being it gives them.

Over the years I've come to realise there are a dozen things we need to help us succeed with regular exercise.

1. **Have a purpose.** Aim for something far enough in the future that it will keep you going for years. It could be wanting to walk 18 holes of golf when you're 85 or living independently in your 90s.

2. **Set a short-to-medium-term goal.** You also want something more readily achievable to keep you going. Maybe you want to look good for your 50th birthday or a university reunion, or maybe you want to have a chance in the parents' race on sports day.

3. **Have a hero to aspire to.** Think of who you'd like to be in the future. That could be a professional athlete, although if so be wary about unrealistic comparisons. It could be someone you know who lives well. I recently heard of a 96-year-old man with an impressive daily exercise routine – touching his toes 100 times, rotating his spine 100 times and doing 100 push-ups off the bar on the Aga, plus taking a 30-second cold shower every morning. He's my inspiration.

4. **Appreciate how fortunate you are.** When I'm running, and my brain tells me to stop (see section on fatigue), I think of how the hospital is full of people who'd love the opportunity to feel the way I'm feeling right now, and that helps me to keep on going to the end. It also helps to remind myself that

I don't have to run for another 48 hours and that that feeling is only temporary.

5. **Link your exercise to an existing task.** Don't spend hours thinking about when you're going to fit your exercise in and only a few minutes actually doing it. A simple trick is to link it to an existing part of your day. I do my core exercise routine when I hang up the washing. It adds 15 minutes to the task but I waste no time procrastinating about it.

6. **Give yourself a carrot.** It's not easy to go out for a run on a cold, wet November night, but that's what it takes to stay on track. Listening to a really good podcast while you work out can be a great incentive, especially if you set a rule to listen only while you exercise. If you can find a podcast that lasts at least the length of three workouts, you'll have another incentive to go out for the next one – plus you might learn a thing or two.

7. **Know who you are and how you think.** Your personality will play an enormous part in your exercise success. If you are disciplined, motivated and appreciative of routine, you'll do all of the above and won't find it too challenging to stay on track. If you aren't, you might need some support from friends who can encourage you to keep going. Joining a group or a class might work better for you, or maybe entering a race or charity event is what you need to keep on keeping on. Perhaps you need a personal trainer to get you to a certain level of fitness before you can go on your own. Think about who you are and how you can work with your strengths when it comes to committing to exercise.

8. **Be accountable.** If you say you are going to do something and write it down, you are 39.5 per cent more likely to succeed

than if you don't put it in writing. If you say you are going to do something and write it down then give that document to someone else, you are 76.6 per cent more likely to succeed.[8] Accountability helps. I will regularly tell patients that I am going for a run later that day, especially when I'm tired or the weather is bad or I simply don't feel like it. I make myself accountable to them and I don't want to be a hypocrite.

9. **Be careful what you measure.** It's easy to fixate on times and performance, but what matters more is that you're exercising – and you're doing it week in, week out. Sure, have an idea of how you are doing so you can see progress and keep motivated, but don't let it ruin your day if you are three seconds slower than your last run. Exercise isn't all about physical performance. Sometimes clearing your head is more important than peak heart rate and split times per kilometre.

10. **Mix it up.** Routine is great but it's easy to get lazy or complacent, so mix it up every now and then. Ask your body some different questions and set yourself some new short-term goals.

11. **Get real.** There are 24 hours in a day and 168 hours in a week. Even if you average an hour a day across all types of exercise, you'll spend less than 8 hours a week exercising. That leaves 160 hours when you're not doing it.

12. **Don't be a passenger.** Life doesn't stop for anyone, but it can certainly pass you by. Take ownership of your health and well-being. You're the one who benefits most and you're the only one who can do something about it.

CHAPTER 6

The Mental Space

THE MENTAL SPACE is your cognitive brain. This is where you use your intellect, stretch yourself cerebrally. For most people, that is their work. Work forms a large part of your identity, how you perceive others see you and how you behave. But very few people work forever and there usually comes a time when you stop doing that role. This can leave a large void in your health hexagon. And yet the mental space isn't just about your job; it includes anything that involves cognitive effort. This could be managing a household, organising your finances, planning for the future, self-improvement or grappling with past trauma.

At times of stress, it's common to bury yourself in the space you are already in, believing that this will solve the problem. If you just get that piece of work done, get that promotion, get that pay rise, finish that report then everything will be OK. You work more hours and ignore your fitness, your sleep, your diet, your family and social life. What actually happens is you eventually finish that piece of work and not only are the other elements of your hexagon out of balance, but another piece of work is likely to come along, so one stress replaces another.

Although we'll mainly be looking at working life in this chapter, the principles are the same for whatever cognitive effort you are dealing with. We will look at purpose, communication, systems, organisation, personality and hierarchy, and options to keep the grey matter working indefinitely. The topics discussed in this section are neither exhaustive nor a prescription. Rather I want to offer some ideas about what might be significant in the mental space. Of course, you can't always assign an activity exclusively to one area; there's usually some overlap. The important thing is to consider the overall effect it has on your health hexagon.

Neurogenesis and clarity of thought

You might expect this chapter to focus on the benefits of exposing your brain to cognitive stimuli. Of course that matters but what most people don't appreciate is that brain function benefits enormously from exercise. Neurogenesis is the process by which the brain grows and replenishes nervous tissue, which helps retain function and memory in the brain. As we get older, the rate of neurogenesis slows down. The turnover rate of new neurons is approximately 1.75 per cent per year in adulthood, accounting for approximately 700 new neurons per day in the hippocampus, which is where a lot of memory is processed.[1]

Exercise has been shown to have enormous neuroprotective and cognitive benefits. Aerobic exercise such as running, cycling, swimming and even having sex has been shown to boost neurogenesis, as does resistance exercise. Mental tasks are important but it seems that a huge effort is necessary to see benefits: learning a new language, for instance, rather than doing yet another crossword or sudoku.[2,3] This might mean that you can most effectively improve your mental agility by working on your physical space.

Studies have shown that speed of thought can improve with exercise: many report having their best ideas as they exercise.[4] Recognising this can allow you to prioritise exercise differently:

going out for a run or a swim or a cycle could be a far more productive way of dealing with a problem at work than sitting in the office for hours. The mental and physical rooms are closely connected: if you set up your life so that exercise is a regular part of it you might discover that you empty that stress bucket more reliably, you organise your thoughts better, you can prioritise problems or challenges more effectively and you are generally more productive and better able to manage stress.

I see so many patients who value their cognitive health far more than their physical health. They understand intellectually that physical activity is important, but it is not as high on their priority list. Once they appreciate the broader benefits of exercise, they are smart enough to understand that they need to introduce this into their life. How they do it is up to them, and I love discovering what works for different people. One highly acclaimed academic I worked with settled on dancing around his kitchen while preparing every meal, snack or cup of tea. As part of his improvised dance routine, he'd do the occasional push-up or squat. Improving your hexagon doesn't necessarily have to involve running marathons.

When you know you have a particularly stressful event coming up or you are dealing with a crisis, it's important to recognise that your cognitive stress bucket is likely to fill up. What can you do to prepare by creating extra capacity?

One patient of mine, Mary, was struggling after her father was diagnosed with Alzheimer's. She lived in a different country and so couldn't provide regular practical help throughout his illness, which caused her a huge amount of guilt. She felt like an imposter who wasn't entitled to an opinion and that other family members viewed her as dropping in from time to time only to fly out again.

She also grappled with a sense of duty, feeling that when she did fly home she ought to spend every minute with her family.

To help her cope with this highly stressful situation, she put various plans into place. Instead of accepting a lift from the airport from a family member, she always hired a car. On landing, she drove first to the beach and went for a short run or walk by the sea, followed by a coffee in a local café. She recognised that a coffee by the sea would do more to empty her stress bucket than a coffee on the plane. The café itself was a welcome break from her reality – full of people going about their seemingly normal day. It was comforting to Mary to be reminded that life goes on regardless – and that you have no idea what others are dealing with as they go about their day.

All of this added 40 minutes to Mary's journey from the airport to the family home. Not an enormous amount of time – but time well spent. When she reached home, she could focus on her dad and have some space to cope. On the drive back to the airport for the return flight she called her partner to offload what had happened, which helped her to process it. None of this removed the stress and anxiety from a very difficult situation, but it gave her a framework to manage it.

Let's look at some ways to take the stress out of the cognitive space.

Purpose

It's essential to have a purpose, by which I mean something to aim for. Something that motivates you and helps stimulate the neurotransmitters that produce feelings of success, confidence, achievement, satisfaction. Some people get this from work while others need to either find a project outside work that gives them that sense of direction and attainment or take a closer look at their job and see where they can find purpose in it.

Let's say you're a bricklayer. Placing brick after brick might feel monotonous after a while, eventually leaving you feeling like you are not doing anything all that special. With that mindset, it's going to be difficult to get through dark, wet, frosty winter mornings. It's going to be harder to put up with the irritations of colleagues, the frustrations of supply issues, a relentless boss, awkward clients, aches and pains and little by way of thanks. But what if your mindset was that you are not just building walls: you are building homes? A place someone has worked to obtain, a place where memories will be made, a construction that really matters. Framed like this, you can take more pride in your work, understanding that you are contributing to something bigger than yourself, and that you are integral to its success.

Many years ago I heard Sir Dave Brailsford speak at a conference about how he had changed the culture of the British Olympic cycling squad to great effect. He spoke of a conversation he had with one of the bike mechanics in his first weeks in his role at Team GB. He pointed out to the mechanic that the wheel he was working on didn't look flush. The mechanic was offended, feeling that he was very experienced at his job and that Brailsford should mind his own business and let him get on with it. After some work on helping all members of the team understand their collective purpose, and the significance of every one of them pulling in the same direction, Brailsford was proud to say that if he were to have the same conversation with the same mechanic now, the mechanic would stop and say, "Where? Show me," so that he could put it right. He no longer saw this as criticism but rather an opportunity to achieve his purpose.

Pursuing your purpose is a great place to be. The painter Fritz Scholder described it as "walking the tightrope between accident and discipline". Working on something that is just beyond your reach challenges you, enabling you to develop new skills and experience. You grow and improve. If something is well beyond your capabilities, that can lead to anxiety or chaos; but if it doesn't challenge you it leads to boredom. And when it comes to boredom, we can learn a little something from rats.

Rat park

Having a purpose is a vital part of seeking fulfilment in life, whatever form that may be. Without it you can easily fall into destructive behaviours. In his TED Talk 'Everything You Think You Know About Addiction Is Wrong', Johann Hari describes Bruce Alexander's "rat park" experiments, which showed what happens when you put a rat in a cage and give it the choice of water or liquidised heroin or cocaine.[5] Rats in isolation with no other stimuli chose the drugs, but when in cages with other rats as well as games or puzzles to pursue, the vast majority avoided them. When they had to learn how to collaborate or establish a place in a hierarchy, when they were challenged, that gave them a truer sense of purpose than the lure of the quick fix.

Without a sense of purpose, each one of us is prone to turning to a quick fix to fill a void. That might be food, alcohol, drugs, shopping, lethargy or gambling. It could be spiralling into office politics or petty squabbles and one-upmanship instead of being able to rise above it. Whether you are working or not, you need something to challenge you cognitively, something to feel proud of, something to give you a reason to stay away from the temptations that will certainly unbalance your hexagon. Purpose is about striving for something bigger than yourself, always giving you something to aim for. But as with everything in your hexagon, you have to figure out what is enough for you – pursuing a particular goal to the exclusion of all else is not a balanced way to live.

If you don't work for an organisation with a clear sense of purpose that you believe in, then you have to find a sense of purpose for yourself. Figure out what sort of wall you are building. Of course, this does not come without its stresses and too much stress is pro-inflammatory, priming your pain system to be hypervigilant. The remainder of this chapter looks at some ways to reduce stress in the workplace, but the principles can be applied to all areas of your life. Perhaps for you, purpose is about being a better parent and spouse while achieving success in your career. This could mean engineering your work in such a way that you can be present for family meals, school performances or sporting events. You can work as a team, so each member of the family feels valued and pulling in the same direction. It's not easy, but if it's consistent with your broader purpose, that will help inspire you to negotiate with the various stakeholders, including yourself, to engineer your hexagon accordingly. That requires the ability to communicate.

A, B, C of communication

It's fair to say that a lot of conflict, and subsequently cognitive stress, comes from poor communication. One of the best pieces of advice I learned on this subject is the four rules of communication, told to me by a patient who had learned them from the head of the Swiss armed forces. The four rules are:

1. Can you hear me?
2. Do you understand me?

3. Do you agree with me?
4. Will you do as I say?

It looks simple, but unless you meet the criteria for all four, you will struggle to get things done or know whether those you are dealing with are in agreement. It's very easy to assume that others share your priorities and that when you speak they are paying attention, but unless you go through each stage in the list you can't know for sure.

It starts with the most basic step. Are you listening to who is talking to you, and are they listening to you? Are you trying to have a conversation with someone while they are busy doing something else, like looking at their phone, typing something or ordering a coffee? You might imagine you can multitask, or they can multitask, but research tells us that it actually takes longer to get things done that way.[6,7] It might feel frustrating to wait for your listener to put their phone down or look up from their desk and give you their full attention, but you won't have to repeat yourself if they are listening in the first place. This goes for all areas of life. How often have you shouted up the stairs at a family member who couldn't hear you over the noise of the hairdryer or the fan in the bathroom or the closed bedroom door when climbing the stairs and getting their undivided attention would have been quicker and less irritating in the long run? Make a conscious effort yourself to give your full attention to others when they are talking to you to reduce the risk of miscommunication. It's a drop or two less in the stress bucket.

Part of improving the mental space in your health hexagon involves consciously creating a culture of respect for your own time. If you know you need to focus on something and you can trust those around you to understand that, you can allocate your time appropriately to both work and other parts of your life. That might mean getting out of the office on time to get to the gym or pick the kids up from school, or to enjoy your walk to catch the train home rather than rushing to get there.

If you can model this consistently, and the people around you understand why, they will see the benefits and a wider culture can develop. You can be available for people, perhaps more than you've ever been, by giving them your full attention when you do communicate with them. This requires discipline, prioritising what is important. What tasks need your full attention so that you can block off time to work uninterrupted on them? Can you create specific time to talk to your team either one-on-one or in regular group meetings or keep periods where your door is open when people can drop in unannounced? Your sense of purpose can help you here, so use it to remind yourself to stay focused on what you need to achieve to enable you to get out of the office on time to have that meal with your family.

My patient Declan told me of a brilliant system he developed with his boss when it came to communication. Over the years they had come to realise that their conversations could be broken down into three categories: A, B or C. An A-type conversation meant "I just need to get something off my chest. I don't need you to offer advice or have an opinion. I just need to be heard". B conversations were defined as: "I've been dealing with this issue. Here's what I'm going to do. I don't need you changing my mind, but you need to be aware of what's happening." Finally, a C conversation was: "I've got this problem, I need your help." They started each meeting by identifying whether it was an A, B or C conversation. Regardless of type, the other would give the speaker their full attention. They might not need to utter a single word in an A conversation, but it was important that the other person was heard. This allowed them to offload issues that were getting on top of them professionally and personally without the other trying to "fix" things unnecessarily.

This can be an effective technique in any relationship. Sometimes you just need to vent, without feeling like you're being fixed or told what to do. It's not always easy to recognise which kind of conversation you are having, but thinking about these types can give you an idea of which space you might be in. When your child starts telling you about something that has upset or frustrated them, try not to jump straight in and fix things. Maybe they need a type A conversation, not a C. You might learn more of what's going on in their life by letting them offload. If your partner comes home from work and starts telling you about a colleague they are having problems with, can you let it roll and ask whether they just need a good old-fashioned rant or would they like your opinion before you jump in to offer it? In a C-type conversation, meanwhile, it's important to understand the other person's point of view before offering your opinion. The simplest way to do this is to summarise it back to them to ensure you do understand what they are trying to say to you.

The next thing to consider is whether you agree with what's being said or not. It's too easy to have a conversation where you avoid speaking up and negotiating for yourself, assuming the other person can somehow read your mind or that an issue will magically resolve itself. Let's say you find yourself agreeing to take on responsibility for a piece of work which deep down you know you don't have capacity to handle on top of everything else. You've just put yourself under more pressure and something somewhere is going to suffer. Instead you need to negotiate for yourself. This might mean saying something like, "Yes, I can do that piece of work; however, if you want me to do that then I won't be able to do these other pieces of work you want me to do also. What is the priority here?" That way you are engaging in the conversation and making sure that when you do agree to something, all parties understand what is involved.

Of course everything involves a bit of give and take. It may well be that you have to take on that piece of work that will put you under pressure, but you negotiate some time or capacity elsewhere at a future date. It might be that you negotiate flexible working hours or an ability to work from home as you get that piece of work done or that you will be able to guarantee time off for some future family event. The key is to go into each conversation with a clear understanding of what you are agreeing to and the consequences it may have for you and those around you.

When agreeing to something you also have to consider your capacity, both at that time and in the future. It's very common to agree to something because at that moment you have some capacity to help. I've seen it time and time again with patients who have taken on a project when they had space but then somewhere down the line three or four projects collide, leaving them over-committed. Then they're back in to see me with a back spasm or tension headache.

Before you agree to something, calculate how the timeline will most likely work out and ask yourself whether you really do have the space. This is as true in life as it is in work. It takes a degree of honesty with yourself and others to realise you cannot be all things to all people, and saying yes or no has consequences. Before you agree to anything, can you ask yourself: Does this align with my purpose, how does it fit into my hexagon, and do I have enough capacity to see it through?

The final part is: Will you do whatever it is you have agreed to or will those around you do whatever it is you think they have agreed to? That comes down to integrity, accountability and an ability to communicate clearly. This requires organisation and having a plan of action for everything you have agreed to do.

Let's take a look at being organised.

Asking the right question

So far, we have considered having clarity of thought, having a sense of purpose, knowing how to communicate and considering what you agree to and how much capacity you have to do it. All of these can help with managing stress events. We can all get stressed when it feels like we have too much to do. We are all busy and often feel pulled in all sorts of directions, so having a way to get things done can reduce the accompanying stress. For many of my patients juggling busy lives, Gary Keller's book *The One Thing* has been a source of great help.

Keller identified that some of the most important things in his life happened as a consequence of making one decision, but he hadn't necessarily considered any of these things before making his decision. For example, when buying a house you'll almost certainly take into consideration what it costs, how many rooms it has, whether you can park your car, if it has a garden, whether it needs much renovation work and how long your commute will be. All important factors to consider. But buying that particular house will also more than likely determine where your kids go to school, who their friends will be, who your friends will be, where you will get your groceries, who your doctor will be, where you exercise and how you socialise, and what community you become a part of. All shaped as a result of buying one house.

Recognising this, Keller came up with his concept of "the one thing". Essentially he asks: What is the one thing I can do that makes everything else easier or unnecessary? He took this approach to many aspects of his life. For example, he wanted to learn to play the guitar from scratch but could devote only 20 minutes a day to doing so as he runs the largest real estate business in the US. The "one thing" he did with his 20 minutes was learn a minor blues scale. Now he can play thousands of songs as a result.

Patients constantly tell me there is no time, but perhaps things don't take as long as you think. Keller's book lays out strategies for developing a "one thing" approach and provides advice on things such as blocking and protecting time, willpower, forming habits and accountability. It can be difficult to figure out what problems need addressing first before you even decide what area your "one thing" question should relate to. The key to a good answer is asking the right question, and it can take some time and consideration to come up with the right answer.

You may need to seek outside help from an expert or a coach when it comes to getting a great answer to your "one thing" question. A new answer usually requires new behaviour. Changing your behaviour can be difficult so it helps to make yourself accountable. Writing down your goals makes you more likely to achieve them. But writing them down and sharing that commitment with someone so you are accountable to them makes you even more likely to succeed.[8] Setting goals and targets and making yourself accountable improves your odds of success, as does committing to spend a certain amount of your time on it. This could involve devoting 20 minutes a week or four hours of your working day – either way it means respecting that time and protecting it.

There will be distractions along the way, whether professional (such as legislative changes, software issues, staff sicknesses and absences, competitors) or personal challenges (unforeseen illness, a family emergency), many of which cannot be foreseen. As you make decisions on projects relevant to your mental space, consider your capacity to cope with the known unknowns alongside any other factors. We'll be thinking about this a little more in the spiritual space chapter.

Mindset

Organising your health hexagon requires a particular kind of mindset. Carol Dweck, author of *Mindset: The New Psychology of Success*, believes there are essentially two types: a fixed mindset and a growth mindset. A fixed mindset is one where you believe that your talents and abilities are fixed in stone. You are either naturally gifted at something, or you are not. Someone with a growth mindset believes that talents and abilities can be developed. Fixed mindsets see every encounter as a test of their worthiness, and in order not to lose status they may avoid challenges. They don't want to look stupid so they won't engage with something where they might fail. A growth mindset individual will see the same encounters as opportunities to improve. They understand that to improve they will inevitably fail along the way. They understand that learning and improving is a lifelong effort, not just reaching a fixed point as defined by a particular exam.

You might have a fixed mindset in certain areas of your life and a growth mindset in others. That's OK – you don't need a growth mindset for everything. But if you want to improve something, you need a growth mindset to do it. To change your mindset, you have to find a cause or a purpose that inspires you. You have to surround yourself with others who you can trust, who you can fail with and who will push you to constantly improve. With a fixed mindset you don't want to look stupid, so you will avoid things where you might fail.

Some of the most successful people I've come across do not mind in the slightest asking questions that to others may look obvious. I had a patient once who was a talented mathematician. He had won the Fields Medal when he was younger, considered one of the highest accolades for a young mathematician. At one point in our conversation, he asked a question that surprised me – it seemed so obvious that the answer was common sense. I remember thinking, This man is a famous mathematician, but he is not the expert in this room and what might be obvious to me is not obvious to him. He has no shame in asking for clarity on something he doesn't understand. This was a pivotal moment for me: no matter how much you do know, you can't know everything, so don't be afraid to ask. It's better to ask a question and "look curious" for a minute than not ask the question and remain ignorant for life.

Personality

We will explore personality in some detail when we enter the emotional space, but at this stage it's worth thinking about how your own personality suits the role you are in or heading towards in your cognitive or mental space.

Imagine a scientist who enjoys his job in a lab, despite the sometimes monotonous tasks involved or the failed experiments. Each has allowed him to inch closer towards enlightenment in the field of research he has dedicated his life to. His devotion to academic excellence has involved long hours in the library, endless research papers. It's been a fairly solitary existence but he is truly passionate about his work and has a real sense of purpose. He worked his way up the hierarchy of their field and now runs a lab that has just made a significant discovery. At this point he is in his sweet spot but the discovery now leads to a crossroads. His institution (this could be a pharmaceutical company or university) wants to showcase the discovery. They want him to network and attend all sorts of social events, conferences and press junkets to promote the organisation. He is incentivised with new titles such as senior fellow or vice president, salary increases, bigger budgets. It seems the logical path to take. His partner, friends, family and colleagues expect it, perhaps already discussing how proud they are of him.

The only problem is he never wanted to be vice president. He hates being paraded about like a trophy. He can no longer do his original job if he's being interviewed endlessly and flying all over the place. This is not his natural habitat and it's leaving him feeling anxious, lost, even depressed. His personality was never a natural fit for such a role and he feels the pressure from those around him, expecting that he should want something that he doesn't want. Society tells us that everyone wants to progress, that happiness lies in getting promoted, higher status, more money. That's how you win the game!

I have seen many high-achieving successful people over the years who have found themselves in this situation. They were passionate about a particular subject and excelled at it. They started a business because they found a question that they wanted to answer. Along the way they discovered that they were no longer purely a scientist or an engineer or a programmer but now a CEO of a business. The more successful their company was and the more employees they had, the more miserable they became and the pain flare-ups increased. They now had board meetings and outside investors calling the shots and they no longer spent much time doing what they loved in the first place. Their success had taken them further away from their sweet spot.

This isn't necessarily a bad thing: success can open other opportunities you may not have anticipated. But if it isn't working for your health hexagon then it can be an opportunity to refocus. For these clients, their new "one thing" became getting "enough" of a fix of their passion to help offset the stresses of running the business. Many decided to block off half a day a fortnight to "play" in the lab. This reinvigorated them and kept them in touch with their passion.

Hierarchy

In the animal kingdom there is a food chain. The lower down that food chain you are, the more predators you have. If you are near the bottom, everything can appear to be a threat. Positions in social hierarchies are closely related to health and disease. Life expectancy in the city of Glasgow can vary by 28 years between the poorest and wealthiest areas of the city.[9] Washington, D.C. has discrepancies of 15 years between some suburbs.[10] Fighting for survival affects your biochemistry and your health. Even when things are plentiful, animal studies from fish to baboons have shown that there is a battle for dominance and subordinates in every group.[11] Research has shown that this has an impact on the levels of serotonin in your brain and this plays a significant role in your confidence and ultimately happiness or contentment.[12] Serotonin also plays a pivotal role in regulating pain (see Chapter 10).

Where you are in any hierarchy can sometimes be objectively determined, but it is also subjective. The scientist in the last section might be considered quite high up the scientific hierarchy, but if he were promoted to vice president of his pharmaceutical company, he might perceive himself at the bottom of the corporate food chain or board-room hierarchy. This could be a welcome challenge if that's the path he wishes to pursue. Or it could cause him to unravel, losing his confidence and feeling like a fish out of water. We've all heard the phrase "a big fish in a small pond". It turns out that the big fish has a different serotonin level to the little fish. Put that big fish in a bigger pond and things might change.

These are the questions you have to ask yourself. Where are you in the food chain? Which hierarchy are you working your way through, and is that the right one for you to focus on? We each exist in many hierarchies for different reasons and different areas of our lives. Perhaps at work you are top of the tree but at home you're very much at the bottom. There may be times when you take a step up only to find it's not the right move for you. That's no bad thing. Now you know where your sweet spot is and you can act accordingly.

Taking everything into account and attempting to balance so many parts of your life seems like an awful lot of work. In fact, it's a lifetime of work because throughout your life where you are in any given hierarchy will change, as will where you are aiming for and where you need to be. In many ways, understanding that is wisdom. Be careful who you compare yourself to and what it is you are comparing. I've seen plenty of patients over the years who would appear to be successful but never feel it. They are always comparing themselves to someone who has in their eyes achieved something bigger or better than they have. A bit of healthy competition with a worthy rival or someone to aspire to can be great for some – but does it work for you? Are you comparing on equal terms? I promise you, no one has it all. It might look like they do sometimes, but they don't. No one wins definitively at life, but it's playing the game that counts, and getting better at playing is where the contentment comes from. Just figure out which games within the game you need to play.

What next? Life after work

I once asked a professional athlete how long he thought he had left in the sport. His answer was: "Sport gives you up, before you give the sport up." Often your work will surpass you. For the athlete, this is when they no longer get picked, their contract isn't renewed, the phone stops ringing – assuming they don't get injured first. When I asked an ageing surgeon a similar question, he assured me that he had trusted colleagues who would tell him when it was time to go. I doubted this very much. It was very unlikely that colleagues would be able to honestly tell him when he was no longer sufficiently competent. That conversation was far more likely to come from the HR department.

One CEO of a large company who had moved multiple times throughout her career told me that an old mentor had advised her to "always leave a job before you grow to resent the good work you've done there". Wise words – though the challenge is knowing when that time approaches.

No matter how important your career is, there is more to you than your job. It's important to consider how you might fill this void when that time comes so it's not a surprise to you when it does. In my job I get to see people through all stages of life.

I believe that curiosity is an essential ingredient to well-being. If you are curious, you will discover a sense of purpose beyond your job, and this will keep you stimulated and give you something to aim for. I know of people in their 80s who struggle to walk because their hip needs replacing, but they still get on their bicycle to get to the library to research their next book or go to a lecture. They are hungry to learn and understand the importance of keeping their mental space occupied with enough stimulus. It would be easy to resign yourself to hip pain and therefore stop moving, but it's amazing what a true sense of purpose can do. I believe you have to work at this mindset – you can't just switch it on when you retire. What you do in each part of your hexagon and how much is enough time to devote to it will change throughout your lifetime, but the principle remains constant.

A friend of mine retired relatively young, in his mid-50s. Over a drink I asked how he was feeling about life post-retirement. He said he had always felt there wasn't enough time in the day and his decision to retire was in part to free up some time to do some of the other things he wanted to do. He was in no way going to be sitting back on his rocking chair for the rest of his days. He had numerous passions to pursue and work on.

The mental space can make your brain hurt, but it also gives you a purpose. If you get this right, you'll be stretching yourself – and who knows what you may find you are capable of. If you get it wrong, you could end up feeling overwhelmed or bored, which can lead to destructive behaviours or drifting into chaos, and that's a pro-inflammatory life. It takes effort to get this balance right. Wherever you find your sense of purpose – in your job, your personal life, your community – you need something meaningful to move towards your whole life.

CHAPTER 7

The Emotional Space

THE EMOTIONAL ROOM is about relationships. Friends, family, colleagues, acquaintances but also about your relationship with yourself – current, past and future. Who you are isn't a fixed destination and every experience you have in life shapes how you think, so it is a constant process of updating.

The people we interact with will have a big impact on how we feel and how we navigate our journey in the world. People can be radiators or drains, filling you with energy or taking it from you. The same people can be both things, depending on how their day is going. Some people are good to be around; others less so. Some people are good to be around sometimes or only for short periods. Everyone is dealing with their own challenges and how their day is going may affect how yours goes too.

Ideally, you should surround yourself with people who want the best for you. This isn't necessarily people who will corroborate your position but will stretch you and challenge you to help you progress along your purpose. Life isn't perfect and you will have to deal with people who are difficult or dangerous and are trying to manipulate you for their own ends. Having enough stimulus in the other areas of your hexagon will help keep your bucket from overflowing.

When it comes to the emotional space your interactions with the people around you matter but so does your perspective. You can't necessarily change how other people will behave, but you can control how you view the situation, which can greatly affect your stress level. For years as a physiotherapist working in professional sport, I used to go on pitch-side first aid courses. One of the skills I had to keep up to date was how to stabilise a spine. That's getting someone safely onto a spinal board where there is a suspicion of a spinal injury, such as after a high-speed collision or a fall from a height.

Ever since I came across this process as an undergraduate, I was terrified of paralysing someone. The slightest movement of their spine and I was sentencing that person to a life of paralysis. I'd been doing these courses for years and years and eventually at the start of one course, the instructor said something that completely changed my perspective: "Remember if they end up paralysed, it's the fall that's paralysed them, not you doing your job … You are there to help stabilise them and as long as you follow your training you are doing everything to help them in that situation."

This completely changed my mindset and helped me see the process in a very different way. In turn that allowed me to be less anxious when working. Rather than dreading the possibility of having to spinal board someone, I trusted my training and realised that if I had to deal with that situation then I could. This didn't change my sense of responsibility and professionalism, or my desire never to have to put those skills into practice, but it did take some emotional stress out of working at such events.

In this section we will look at the two things that have the greatest impact on the emotional space: your personality and the personalities of everyone else you deal with. We will also look at family dynamics, peer groups and a couple of neurotransmitters. Before we do that, let's explore some of the science behind stress.

Stress and the hypothalamic-pituitary-adrenal axis

The hypothalamic-pituitary-adrenal or HPA axis is a complex neuroendocrine system that helps regulate many body processes such as mood, emotions, energy storage, the digestive system, the reproductive system, the cardiovascular system, the metabolic system and the immune system.[1]

When stimulated, a part of the brain called the hypothalamus secretes two peptides called vasopressin and corticotropin-releasing hormone (CRH). These regulate the anterior lobe of the pituitary gland in the brain and together stimulate adrenocorticotropic hormone (ACTH). ACTH then stimulates the cortex of the adrenal gland, which sits above the kidneys and produces glucocorticoid hormones. In humans this is mainly cortisol, which is made from cholesterol. As levels of these glucocorticoids rise in the bloodstream, they in turn act back on the hypothalamus and pituitary to suppress the production of CRH and ACTH, ideally switching off the stress response once it's dealt with.

The hypothalamus releases CRH in response to stress, physical activity and illness and at various stages of the sleep-wake cycle (circadian rhythm). The HPA axis combines physical and psychological stresses to adapt to your environment so you can use your resources effectively to survive. If you're being chased by a fierce animal or crossing a road while a car comes towards you, the stress of that situation will activate your HPA axis. Your body releases cortisol, which will mobilise glucose stores and stimulate blood flow away from your digestive system into your legs to give you a boost of energy to get out of danger. Digesting your lunch is not a priority at that moment! Cortisol will also suppress the immune system, which uses up a lot of energy, therefore making more glucose available if you need it to react to the immediate danger.

In excess cortisol can be damaging and has been linked to atrophy of the hippocampus, which is an important part of the brain in memory and formulating an appropriate response to stress.[2] In Chapter 11 we will look in more detail at the various centres of the brain and their specific roles, but for now it's worth pointing out that the amygdala also has connections with the HPA axis. The amygdala looks out for threats. If it perceives something to be dangerous, it will activate the HPA. Similarly, if the HPA is already activated the amygdala will become more alert to danger. This is important when it comes to persistent pain and stress as a trigger. Your stressors will be different from other people's and the activation of your HPA axis will depend on your tolerance for fear and resilience to stressors.

As our brains develop so does our tolerance for stress. Early-life stresses seem to influence the sensitivity of the HPA axis. In animal models, mild to moderate early stressors enhance HPA regulation, building some lifelong resilience to stress. Having a less than "perfect" childhood could be helpful in the long run. Our bones respond to load-bearing by getting stronger – but too much can cause stress fractures, and it appears the HPA system may work similarly. Early exposure to extreme or prolonged stress can result in a hyperreactive HPA axis and may contribute to lifelong vulnerability to stress.[3,4] Adult victims of childhood abuse for instance have shown higher levels of ACTH in response to psychological stress.[5] Early life stress can sensitise the HPA axis, resulting in a particularly heightened response to stress-induced CRH.

With repeated exposure to stress, the sensitised HPA axis may continue to secrete CRH from the hypothalamus, contributing to anxiety symptoms. There is some evidence that prenatal stress during pregnancy can affect HPA axis excitability in humans, and some studies have found an association between maternal depression and altered cortisol levels in early childhood.[6,7] This all happens before you have any conscious control over it and contributes to the hand you are dealt or your default setup. Having some insight into your tolerance for stress or the excitability of your HPA axis can help you prioritise activities that help regulate your HPA axis when considering your health hexagon. There is evidence that an increase in the neurotransmitter oxytocin, which we get from positive social interactions, helps suppress the HPA axis and therefore counteracts stress. We will look at other activities that impact your HPA axis in due course.

The sensitivity of our stress response systems can be affected by a wide variety of circumstances: simply growing up in a time of distress or uncertainty can have an influence. An experiment involving primates can help explain this. In this experiment infants were growing up with what would be considered normal maternal care. Each mother and infant were put into one of three groups where the mother had to forage for food. In group one it was consistently easy to find food and therefore easy for the mother monkey to look after her infant. In group two it was consistently difficult to find food, and in the third group it was random – sometimes easy, sometimes difficult. The researchers observed the nature of the mother-infant relationships during the test period, the personality traits developed by the infants, and the biochemical status of the young monkeys' stress systems throughout their lifetime.[8]

In the groups where it was consistently easy or difficult to find food, the mother monkeys did not seem to experience either as a stressful situation. The variable conditions, however, created a stressful environment for the mothers. These mothers exhibited "inconsistent and erratic, sometimes dismissive, rearing behaviour". The infants grew up to be anxious, less social and highly reactive to stressful situations as adults. This groups of monkeys had lifelong elevated levels of corticotropin-releasing hormone (CRH) in their cerebrospinal fluid, indicating an excitability in their stress apparatus.

It's important to remember that the mothers didn't reject their infants and that the mothers in the other two groups weren't "better" parents; rather the unpredictability of the environment of the third group was a physiological and psychological stressor. The environment contributed to a situation where the parent was physically but not necessarily psychologically present. This is known as proximate separation and the physiological stress experienced by a child in this situation approaches the levels experienced during physical separation.[9]

In his book *In the Realm of Hungry Ghosts*, psychiatrist Gabor Maté explains how such situations disrupt the development of the brain's neurotransmitters and self-regulation systems and in particular the stress control circuits. This sort of physiological dysfunction increases the risk for addictive behaviours. Both animals and humans use substances or behaviours to modulate their experiences of stress.[10] This might include drugs, alcohol or eating; activities such as shopping, gambling, sexual promiscuity or excessive exercise; or behaviours like perfectionism, obsessional behaviour and rigidity in routines. It could also be jumping from fad to fad, chasing a buzz that quickly fades, each time replaced by a new craze within a few years or months.

Bringing up children today, increasingly without the historical support of a tribe, community or extended family, presents increasing challenges that can make it difficult for parents to be present emotionally for their children as their brains develop. I see many patients with deep-seated issues with their parents, heavily influencing their thinking and leaving them struggling to move forward. They get trapped in chaos. Often the problem may not have started with them. Their ability to be a parent is influenced by their own upbringing and development and the generations and generations before them. They may not have had the skills or resources to cope either. No one has a perfect childhood, but each of us can do something about our future.

Just as your upbringing will be unique to you, so is your brain development, the sensitivity of your stress system and your personality. Everyone has "gaps" in their development. As we go through life, we gravitate towards behaviours that regulate or fill these gaps.[11] In some sense we are all addicted to something to try to balance the neurochemical physiology of the consequences of our upbringing. This isn't necessarily dysfunctional in and of itself, but some strategies are more helpful than others.

Personality

By having better insight as to who you are, you can understand a bit more about how you react to the world and situations around you. Each personality trait has its strengths and weaknesses and the diversity of combinations of personality traits in the human race is what makes the world go around.

We need different people with different skill sets and different points of view to fulfil different roles and come up with new ideas. There is much evidence in the workplace that diversity helps improve and progress things. It can be straightforward to think about diversity along the lines of gender, race, ethnicity, sexuality, disability and religion, but it is also about mindset and thinking: two people who look the same can be very different in how they view the world.

We can learn skills to cope with particular situations. Do you remember the scientist in the mental space who was more introvert than extrovert? He felt more comfortable with fewer people and was uncomfortable in situations where he needed to network with lots of different people and "sell" himself. Provided he doesn't have to do this too often, that he believes that such networking will help towards their purpose, and that he has enough capacity in his stress bucket to cope with this scenario, he can manage for a short time. He might be out of his comfort zone, but he can cope with this challenge in his emotional space provided he has enough capacity from the other parts of his hexagon. This might include physical exercise to help with clarity of thought, emotional support from trusted colleagues, mentors or partners to reassure him that it will be OK, he can do it and these colleagues will act as allies and give him an excuse to leave should they see he is getting too anxious. He might use breathing techniques from the spiritual space or an internal meditative mantra such as "tomorrow I'll be in my lab, and this allows me to be there".

But if he's under stress and he hasn't used his hexagon to give him that capacity to cope, he is more likely to revert to his default personality setting, perhaps even going a little further into introversion. He's likely to find it more difficult to cope with a challenge like networking and he might start experiencing anxiety, maybe even pain. The important thing in using your hexagon to cope with stress is to build a routine that empties that stress bucket regularly and reliably so that you have capacity to cope in the future. You have to build that reliable routine and put it into practice regularly, not just on the day of the stressor, so that you have the capacity to deal with these situations.

The Big Five Aspect scale takes five personality traits and sub-divides each into two components:

1. Agreeableness: compassion and politeness
2. Conscientiousness: industriousness and orderliness
3. Extraversion: enthusiasm and assertiveness
4. Neuroticism: withdrawal and volatility
5. Openness to experience: openness and intellect

Depending on the situation, your personality settings can be adjusted slightly up or down. For example, you might have a very different attitude towards orderliness when you are on holiday as compared to when you are at work. At the start of a holiday, when you are still in work mode and your stress bucket is full, if you score high in orderliness (an aspect of conscientiousness), you might get very frustrated with a messy hotel room. By the time you are a few days into your holiday and your stress bucket is emptying, you might be less bothered and can close the door and go out and enjoy your holiday. In a work setting, however, it might be that you can't think clearly unless everything is neat and tidy. At home you might not be able to relax if one room is untidy, even if you are not in it. Knowing this about yourself can help you realise why you might be feeling irritated about something, and that knowledge can be extremely useful.

Your personality traits have consequences for those you live and work with. If your partner is just a little lower on the scale for orderliness than you are, you are likely to get frustrated by something that is not in order about 20 seconds sooner than they do. You are likely to tidy things up first even though they would do it too if you left it a little longer. Because you react first, you feel like you are always the one tidying up while everyone else is lazy.

It doesn't take a huge discrepancy on a given trait scale to have an impact on your behaviour and how you feel. The important thing to remember is that when you are under stress you default back to your settings, and that 20 seconds could be the difference between getting very frustrated or not. If you find yourself feeling this way, acknowledging that you might be defaulting to your trait setting and are struggling to regulate yourself, you can use one of the other parts of your hexagon to deal with it. Your trait settings are pretty difficult to completely adjust. Generally you can nudge them a bit but not reverse them – at least, not without a great deal of effort and purpose.

When I did the Big Five Aspect scale questionnaire,* I scored low for agreeableness. Initially when I saw the report I was offended; I thought I was a reasonably agreeable person. It took me a little time to digest the information in context. Men typically score lower on the agreeableness scale than women. I scored highly in trait intellect, which is a measure of interest in abstract thinking and not to be confused with intelligence. I was

---

* See for example www.understandmyself.com.

lower than average in enthusiasm and high in assertiveness. This combination suggests I tend to think through a process quickly and that I don't get terribly excited about things if I don't feel they are all that important at the time; and my assertiveness means I tend to put my opinion across strongly. This became clearer to me when my wife suggested we get some new sofas.

She made the suggestion on a Friday evening when my head was still in work mode, and I essentially shot it down straight away. I had defaulted to my agreeableness setting and didn't let her go through her process of thinking out loud, which is how she likes to work through something. The reason I said no was because I knew she hadn't decided what sofa she wanted. I knew the type of sofa was more important to her than it was to me and that ultimately she would be the one making the decision. I also knew that we might spend half a dozen weekends going around sofa shops without making a purchase and that this would be difficult to juggle alongside the children's sports, homework and various birthday parties, never mind trying to get some exercise in ourselves, cut the lawn, do the food shopping and have the odd lie-in. My higher-than-average scoring for orderliness meant I needed to be on top of the logistics, and window shopping for sofas didn't fit in with that plan. For me.

When I did the personality test and told her I was low on agreeableness, her reaction was unsurprising: "You don't say!" Now that I understand this about myself, if I shoot something down without giving it a fair hearing my wife will say, "How's your agreeableness?" I'll acknowledge that and say, "Fair enough; can we talk about this tomorrow?" It tells me I must be under some stress without necessarily having realised it and that another time of day might be better for us to talk about something.

I've also tried to practise this at work and among friends where I hear myself ready to jump in and shoot something down. Instead, when I can, I try to nudge that agreeableness dial just a touch and let things run. Where I've learned to identify that some people like to think out loud and walk and talk their way through an issue, I can now see that I need to let that happen. Just as with the rules of communication – maybe they want an A-type conversation and they are not actually asking me for anything.*

The information gathered from such a profiling tool is complex and this book is not about breaking that down. I am simply making the point that your personality will play a large role in how you feel and engage with the world and those around you. Certain trait combinations can lead to tendencies towards certain behaviours. If you score average in conscientiousness and high in neuroticism, you may well have a tendency towards procrastination. If you are high in intellect but low in industriousness, you are likely to come up with good ideas but will need help with supervision and accountability. If you are high in openness but low in conscientiousness and high in neuroticism, you will learn quickly and be creative but have difficulty implementing your ideas.

Greater insight into yourself can help you put the necessary processes in place to help you achieve your purpose, find that sweet spot in a hierarchy and regulate the neurotransmitters that determine which bus you take on your pain pathway. If you need help being conscientious, look for someone who will mentor you and hold you accountable. Recognise where your personality is

---

* We got new sofas in the end. My wife spent hours looking online and decided what she wanted. When she did, she said, "I think I like this one, shall we go and look at it?" We did. We liked it. We bought two. It took about 30 minutes.

a strength and where it is a weakness, and where you can put a system or structure in place to help.

As with the physical space, you may need the support of a friend or a professional to help you commit to your goals. You need to surround yourself with people who want the best for you and can nudge those personality traits to help you be a more rounded individual. Animals find a niche within an environment that matches their skill set. Polar bears don't live in the Amazon for a multitude of reasons. We need to take a similar approach when it comes to our unique personalities and tolerance for stress. We need to find the environment and the support that helps us best to thrive.

Now let's take a look at everyone else.

Other people

No one is an island. No matter how much you might isolate yourself, you still need other people. Gaining a better understanding of other people and how they might think will help you communicate and negotiate with them. The clashes that occur as a result of contrasting beliefs and behaviours can be a source of stress and frustration. Persistent pain is stimulated by stress. Short periods of stress are fine but sustained exposure has consequences for your biochemistry and your well-being.

A patient once told me about his work on an oil rig. It's a difficult environment – a bunch of men in a confined isolated space working in tough conditions for six weeks at a time. Finding ways to minimise conflict is essential. On my patient's rig, all employees had to wear different coloured hard hats to represent how they behaved under stress. Everyone was educated on what the various colours meant. Some people under stress would get loud and shout and swear, others would go quiet, some would get really chatty, and some might become physically aggressive. Knowing how someone behaved under stress allowed them to better understand their co-workers' behaviour during difficult times. They could then understand when a problem wasn't necessarily with them but with their co-worker. It gave people insight into themselves and allowed them to moderate their own behaviour, but it also took some of the heat out of an intense situation.

The popular book *Surrounded by Idiots* by Thomas Erikson has been enlightening in identifying different personality profiles: How different people think, how they behave under stress and how to negotiate with different personality types. Understanding yourself is useful; understanding that other people don't see the world the way you do gives you some insight into how and why your stress buttons can be pushed by certain people in certain scenarios. This understanding can help you shift your perspective on where they are coming from, meaning those buttons don't get pushed as readily.

Venn family

I've come to realise that families are like a Venn diagram. We start off in one circle as a family unit, parents and siblings. Over time additional people come into the family, such as partners. If you have children, you start your own circle. As your new circle influences your thinking, you may find that what you have in common with your original family circle diminishes. As other siblings do the same thing, the overlap between the original family unit can get smaller and smaller.

Over time, your outlook on life tends to change. As you grow older it's very possible that the way you see the world and moderate your behaviour is now very different from that of your childhood self. But when you are thrown back into the original family circle, it's not uncommon to revert to your original role within the family pecking order. This can feel at odds with your present self, which often leads to frustration. The challenge is in recognising that this is normal. Different people want different things from their lives and the close relationship perhaps that siblings once had will likely take on a different nature. These dynamics have to be redrawn as circumstances change, as people move to different areas of their lives and have different needs and aspirations.

There is usually common ground, but it takes a bit of work to figure out where that is. It might look different for individuals within the family dynamic such as mother-daughter, father-son, brother-sister and every combination in between. The art is to find the common ground in each of those relationships and within the whole. As always, it's a question of balance. I see numerous patients who suffer pain flare-ups around family events. If you're spending too much time pushing yourself into stressful territory, you need the tools to help offset such stresses. That's where the health hexagon can help.

A common family stressor crops up when it comes to child-care. If you're a grandparent, the idea of helping your children and spending time with your grandchildren may sound like a brilliant idea – and of course it can be if everyone finds the sweet spot where it works. But don't forget to ask yourself, What is enough? People are having children later and later and grandparents are older and older. I see plenty of people in their 70s with persistent back and neck pain because they are just not able to cope with the volume of childcare they are doing. Early starts and the constant vigilance involved in looking after babies and toddlers is physically and mentally exhausting, never mind the potential clashes in parenting styles and values.

It's important to think carefully about what you are letting yourself in for as a grandparent and whether you have capacity in your physical and emotional bucket for it. If your parents are looking after your child while you work, do you know what you are expecting of them and how this might stretch the dynamics in the family as a whole? It can be very difficult for a grandparent to say they can't cope – if so, their pain system might need to draw their attention to the problem.

Crisis? What crisis?

If you are feeling stretched in your emotional space, it's easy to get overwhelmed by a problem. A crisis can feel all-consuming. It helps as always to have a sense of perspective. What feels like a crisis to you can be another day in the office for someone else, and sometimes it helps to appreciate that your crisis is not a crisis for everyone else. We can only deal with a situation with the tools we have available. If you don't have the correct tools to cope or if you're not sure which tools to deploy, stepping out from a crisis to get the perspective of someone else, someone with some experience, can be essential.

Late one Friday afternoon I received an email from the company I use for our clinic practice management software "reminding" me that the software I was using would be discontinued at the end of the month and I wouldn't have access to our database in three weeks. This came as a massive surprise as it was brand-new information to me. It was also a couple of weeks before Christmas and the thought of sourcing new software, transferring

THE EMOTIONAL SPACE

all the clinic information, training staff and making sure appointments and finances were all in order for the new year was not what I had planned to do with the Christmas period. It would have been very easy to bury myself in this crisis, spending hours and hours researching software companies and cancelling all other activities. Instead, I followed my health hexagon and played golf as I had planned to on Saturday morning.

Ordinarily my mind would have been on the golf and perhaps a degree of anxiety over how well I would play. That morning what mattered most was to get out on the course and clear my head so I could approach my work crisis with some logic and a degree of distance. Halfway up the first hole one of my playing partners asked me how work was going. I explained the unexpected email I had received, and his reaction was so calm and neutral it was very reassuring. He had recently retired and his response to my crisis was, "I remember those days. That's really frustrating."

It turned out that was what I needed: someone not emotionally involved in the situation to say the equivalent of "Yeah, that's rubbish, but it comes with the territory – and don't worry, you can handle it. Look at me, I'm out on the golf course with all of that behind me and your 'crisis' will be a distant memory someday too." He gave me a sense of direction with his reminder that one day all those work frustrations would be behind me. It was a bump in the road, not the end of the world, and although I wasn't expecting it, that's life.

That 20-second conversation helped me realise that all the permutations that were going through my head of how this might play out and the frustrations that fixing it would involve were part of running a business. I knew this anyway but it's important to be reminded. I was getting stressed about the prospect of my clinic looking disorganised to others and whether, if the practice management software wasn't perfect, there would be confusion come the new year. Rather than jumping 50 steps ahead with an emotional bias, I needed to clear my head and look at it logically and practically.

Knowing you are not alone and that other people have experienced what you are going through really helps. Other people can provide reassurance if you've never experienced a particular situation before and so don't know if what you are feeling or doing is normal or the right way to approach things. Practical counsel from someone who's been through what you're now facing helps – whether that's bereavement, relationship breakdown, coping with sick children, trauma or an unexpected IT issue.

A crisis can also be an opportunity. I've known numerous patients who run a business or manage a team and think they are indispensable. One day they get injured or sick and they can't get into the office. They are forced to delegate or let others rise to the challenge. It doesn't always work out, but often they are pleasantly surprised. A business can survive without you for a bit. Sometimes people will step up and prove themselves and maybe you could let them do it sooner rather than waiting for the inevitable crisis to force your hand.

Peer support

Finding a peer group also helps through tough times. High achievers can struggle with this. If you are at the top of a hierarchy then it isn't always obvious who your peers are and you may have to think a little laterally to find that group. Mentoring and coaching are common in lots of fields of life and successful people understand the value of this, but sometimes you need empathy and understanding. There is a great solace in knowing you are not alone, no matter how isolated you may feel. This is what a peer group can offer but it needs to be safe and somewhere that you can be vulnerable. Often when you are at the top of the hierarchy, you cannot allow yourself to show vulnerability.

It might look like a group of business owners who can speak freely to each other without being direct competitors. It might be a bunch of new dads dealing with the loss of their old identity now that they are fathers. It could be a group of female medical consultants who are heads of different departments in different hospitals. Whatever it is, there is huge value to finding a group of people who can empathise with what you're going through as they are going through a form of it too.

Many of my patients are high achievers and have reported struggling to find a peer group or didn't appreciate they needed one until they found it. They have friends or colleagues, partners or coaches and mentors that they talk to, but no one they consider to be their professional equivalent. This isn't arrogance; rather it reflects the fact that some people attain positions that are so few and far between it's difficult to have an equivocal peer. I'm thinking of the likes of a female board member in a very male-dominated industry. It's likely to be difficult to find someone else who may be juggling being on the board of a testosterone-fuelled business while breastfeeding at the same time.

If you've been more successful than your family members and friends, who are your peers? Who can you trust within your organisation or industry? Where can you be vulnerable and speak freely about your concerns and how it feels to be you? Spouses and partners can offer an empathetic ear, but they may not know what it's like to be you at work. In a suitable peer group, you can share the burden of your job. It's important to know that other people feel like you do and understand your challenges or share in your successes without feeling guilty or embarrassed about them. We need to offload those feelings to empty the stress bucket a little, and empathy helps.

As with everything in the health hexagon, enough is key. You don't have to be in each other's pockets for a peer group to be effective. Enough might be meeting for lunch or dinner once every couple of months. But that lunch might be every bit as important as the board meeting or the gym or a night's sleep so it is worth planning and committing to such dates regularly.

People in persistent pain often feel that they are unique as nothing works for them in terms of treatment and it seems that medical experts can't offer answers that make sense. Online forums full of people offering opinions can be alluring in such situations, but those opinions may not be right for you and could even be dangerous. A reliable peer group is likely to prove more useful. The number of people overcoming and managing persistent pain is growing so keep yourself open to looking out for them. When you find them, engage in a conversation and see if you can establish that healthy peer group.

When I worked in professional horse racing, I was surrounded by people obsessed with weight. It's part of their job and the culture of the sport. I began weighing myself daily and being much more conscious than I had ever been before about weight. I didn't think my behaviour was unusual as I was surrounded by people being weighed numerous times a day and conversations about weight were commonplace. As a physio dealing with jockeys, I was inevitably fuelling those conversations too. When jockeys are "doing light", they are down to their minimum allowable weight.

This essentially means they will be dehydrated. They are likely to have stiff, sore joints and muscles as a consequence. This is helpful to know when assessing and treating them, but as a result you are asking them about their weight all the time.

A conversation I had with one jockey who had broken his ankle opened my eyes to the unhealthy relationship jockeys tend to have with weight. When he came out of his cast, I measured the muscle bulk of both ankles and explained that they had lost the equivalent of a couple of centimetres of muscle. Most athletes are anxious about this sort of thing as it can represent a threat to their fitness and ultimately career. Assuming he would be a bit frustrated, I reassured him that it would all be good in the end. I'd help him regain his muscle bulk through the rehab and it wouldn't affect his career long-term. His reaction was not quite what I expected. He said: "Muscle is heavier than fat, isn't it? Great, a couple of centimetres. That means I can have breakfast!"

That relationship with weight and food was very different to mine and I realised that being around that culture long enough risked changing my view of normal. Behaviour can start to creep in which can seem normal in one cohort of people, but is it really healthy for you? It's important to stay alert to the culture of a group and whether it aligns with your purpose.

Who you should trust is not always obvious, and it can get complicated with friends and family. I call this "the Gladys effect". A medical consultant I know had this challenge with her mother. It's fair to say the consultant knows a thing or two about illness and disease. Her mother is a wonderful woman but would rather trust her friend Gladys than her daughter when it comes to medical matters. Gladys is lovely and she makes great cakes, but her knowledge of medicine is limited by comparison. Although her mother is immensely proud of her daughter, at some level she's still the child and Gladys is the grown-up.

A couple of neurotransmitters

Your emotions will depend in part on the balance of neurotransmitters in your brain. We know that anxiety and mood disorders are influenced by serotonin, dopamine, norepinephrine and GABA (γ-aminobutyric acid) among others.[12] Broadly speaking, a family of anti-depressants called SSRIs work by reducing the reuptake of serotonin in the brain, meaning that the prolonged presence of serotonin may help reduce the symptoms of depression and improve your sense of confidence.

Oxytocin is the neurotransmitter of safety, attachment and empathy. It is involved in forming a bond between mother and child, between sexual partners, between owners and their pets. It helps in modulating fear and anxiety and there is some evidence that it may have promise as an anti-depressant and even in reducing some inflammatory cytokines that may contribute to the rate of wound healing.[13] Balancing your health hexagon involves nurturing your relationships, recognising that those around you need your support as much as you need theirs.

We all need to feel safe and secure, and serotonin and oxytocin help us feel this way. This is not just a nice idea; it's biology. Organising your emotional space and balancing the other parts of your hexagon helps keep stress, anxiety, low mood and pain at bay. These feelings have their purpose. They can alert you when something needs adjusting in your hexagon. They remind you of what's working and what isn't. The problem is when they take over.

The emotional space is how you feel. How you feel is grounded in your biology, your genetics, your brain development, the environment you grew up in, the people you grew up with, your tolerance for stress and the experiences you have along the way, as well as the situations you put yourself in, how you perceive them and how you handle them. How you negotiate for yourself and what purpose you find for yourself. Your behaviour will be influenced by your core values and attitude, which you then moderate to suit the situation you find yourself in. If you understand the strengths and weaknesses of your personality, you can carve out a path that harnesses them to the best effect. Stress, contributing to a pro-inflammatory lifestyle, comes in where you don't have the skills or capacity to cope with the situation you find yourself in and when you can't moderate your behaviour appropriately to that situation.

Next up in your health hexagon, you need opportunities to be yourself. You need opportunities to get lost, to play and explore.

CHAPTER 8

The Spiritual Space

IN THE EMOTIONAL ROOM we talked about having to moderate behaviour to deal with the various people and situations in your life. This can be exhausting, and you need time to take off the various masks you wear and just be yourself every now and again. Generally speaking, the spiritual room is the one most people neglect because it feels indulgent, or due to perceived lack of time. But if you spend too much time pushing yourself in stressful situations, you need to recalibrate. Exercise can be great, but there are only so many miles you can run or push-ups you can do, and more isn't always better. Offloading to trusted friends helps, but sometimes you may not have the energy or inclination to talk, or they may not be available. Sometimes you just need space to be yourself.

The spiritual room is that transcendental space where you are lost in the moment. Nothing else matters and you can escape from the stresses and frustrations that otherwise encroach on your thinking. You might not recognise what you are doing as spiritual and that's fine – it can occur in many forms. Mindfulness, for example, is about being fully present and aware of where you are and what you are doing – it could involve allowing yourself to experience the sensation of sunlight on your face or notice your lungs filling with air. There is some evidence that meditation practice can help reduce anxiety, depression and pain.[1] It could be playing sport or a completely different hobby; it could be socialising with friends and getting absorbed in a conversation or attending a concert or play; it could be something creative like painting, baking or gardening.

Whatever it is, the main thing is that it allows you to be fully present in what you are doing, free from distraction. This might seem like the first thing to fall by the wayside when life is busy, but enough time doesn't have to be much time.

Take a breath in the shower

Breathing comes so naturally that it's easy to disregard its importance. It's not only about oxygenation. We've all seen the movies where a character hyperventilating is given a brown paper bag to breathe into to help them calm down. Pausing to take a deep breath when you're feeling tense or frustrated can help you gather your thoughts, while breathing techniques used during labour can help reduce the pain of childbirth. A yawn or a large sigh are autonomic methods your body uses to regulate its oxygen intake. Under stress or tension, apical or thoracic breathing is common: this involves short, shallow breaths rather than deep diaphragmatic breathing. Most people won't even recognise they are doing it. Rarely do people set some time aside to check in with their breathing or practise breathing techniques for relaxation, but it could be a very quick win for your spiritual space.

A number of breathing techniques have been shown to have benefits for relaxation and anxiety reduction. They include alternative nostril breathing, belly breathing, four square breathing, 4-7-8 breathing, lion's breath, mindful breathing, pursed-lip breathing, resonance breathing and more.[2] Deep and slow breathing techniques have been shown to influence pain perception and improve mood by reducing tension, anger and even depression.[3]

You will be familiar with that sharp intake of breath that comes with jumping into cold water or turning on a shower that is colder than you expected. That sudden sharp intake of breath is an autonomic reaction, which is part of your fight-or-flight system. It turns out that a voluntarily induced shock, such as immersing yourself in cold water or consciously induced cycles (three sessions) of hyperventilation (30–40 deep breaths in a row) followed by long periods of holding your breath (90 seconds to three minutes), could be good for training your stress response system. Dutch athlete Wim Hof has gained the nickname "The Iceman" along with 21 Guinness World Records for feats of extraordinary human endurance. He has climbed Kilimanjaro in his shorts, swam under ice for 66 m, ran a half marathon above the Arctic Circle barefoot and popularised cold showers as a way of managing stress and staying healthy. He also developed a technique called the Wim Hof Method: it involves meditation, breathing techniques and exposure to cold, and is starting to gain a significant amount of scientific interest for its potential to influence the autonomic nervous system and innate immune system.[4]

A number of studies have been carried out over the past decade looking into this method and its effect on naturally occurring proteins called interleukins that are known to be involved in the inflammation system. It seems that his method can activate the sympathetic nervous system, increasing anti-inflammatory interleukins and lowering pro-inflammatory ones.[5,6] If you're interested in the science behind the Wim Hof Method, there are various digestible lessons available online.[7,8,9]

A study by Geert A. Buijze and colleagues in the Netherlands looked at 3,018 participants aged between 18 and 65 years old. For 30 days they had their normal hot shower every morning followed by either 30, 60 or 90 seconds of a cold shower between 10 and 12 degrees C. The study was looking at the effect cold showers had on sickness absence. On average across the groups those who took cold showers every day had 29 per cent fewer absent days from work; if they combined this with regular exercise, they had 54 per cent fewer absences in comparison to controls.[10] It turns out there was no difference between 30, 60 or 90 seconds so a quick blast of cold water for 30 seconds every morning could boost your immune system, and you'll probably take a few deep breaths while you're at it.

If hyperventilation and cold showers aren't quite for you, there are plenty of other ways to reduce stress. Maybe instead you'd prefer to play.

Play and palliative care

Palliative care nurse Bronnie Ware famously compiled a list of the top five regrets expressed by her patients in the last days and weeks of their lives. Number one on that list was "I wish I'd had the courage to live a life true to myself, not the life others expected of me."

Life is a matter of negotiation and compromise. Few people are successful enough to live a life true to themselves without having to sacrifice something in life. Unfortunately many, if not most, of us compromise more than is good for us and end up living a life in conflict with who we are designed to be. You try to conform to a version of yourself that others expect of you, or that you perceive to be expected of you. The classic scenario is where a young person is shepherded to a particular career such as doctor or lawyer or in times past a nun or priest because it was considered a reliable, secure, high-status or honourable route to take. If that is not what you ever desired for yourself and you couldn't or didn't speak up, you will probably feel like you are wearing a mask most of the time. You have invested too much time and energy into fulfilling that role; others rely on you to sustain it; and you feel trapped.

Play allows you to explore those other facets of yourself. Children do this all the time when they play. They try out different personas to see how they feel, and they get a sense of whether they might like them. They test one, they test how others react to it. They tweak it a bit and eventually discover what they like, what they don't like, where they fit in and where they don't. As a grown-up, you need opportunities to do this too. Such play allows you to try a different role and if you like it, perhaps find the courage to change direction. Or maybe you discover that it wasn't all it was cracked up to be and achieve a peace with having dipped your toe in the water. Maybe by playing in that role it gives you enough stimulus in that space to offset wearing a mask elsewhere. Hobbies or volunteering can offer this. The world is full of amateur dramatics groups, choirs, singers, musicians, dancers, painters, sculptors, hobbyists, volunteers, local politics, charities, clubs and societies, boards of governors, officers in organisations and countless sporting bodies – all offering opportunities to get a taste of a life you might have had and could have. The rise of the gig economy also offers opportunities to test things out for size, playing at different careers before picking a direction of travel.

Taking that to another level, the concept of deep play involves a degree of risk; it is even potentially life-threatening in order to develop survival skills and conquer fear. For children this might be climbing a tree or standing up to a bully. As we get older the activities become riskier: climbing a mountain, parachuting, hang-gliding, swimming with sharks. Deep play usually involves exposure to the elements and speaks to our ancient need to explore.

The ancient Chinese philosophy of yin-yang, represented by a black and white swirl within a circle with a spot of each contained within the other, symbolises opposite forces interconnected and counterbalancing each other. Order contains a little bit of chaos, offering mystery and adventure into the unknown and ensuring that things are not too safe; chaos contains a little bit of order, offering hope and stability when things become overwhelming. Can you tread the line between the two, finding that sweet spot where you can challenge yourself enough to give your life some meaning and purpose, and ultimately contentment?

Play of some description, whether that be sport, a creative hobby such as art, baking, music or gardening, meditation, mindfulness, deep play or otherwise, provides an opportunity to give order to your chaos or some chaos to your order. As always, it's about enough stimulus for you so you can balance out the other parts of your hexagon. Some people need to climb a mountain and others do it by completing a jigsaw or lying on a hammock looking at the sky.

Hobbies or play can give you that warm, fuzzy feeling of having something to get you through the dark wet winter nights or the slow drudgery of the tasks you don't enjoy. Having something to aim for or complete like rehearsing for a concert or finishing a painting or DIY project helps, as many aspects of life can feel endless. Completing something provides a sense of achievement, closure, satisfaction and relief. Many patients I see feel like their work in particular is endless. Despite being objectively success-ful they feel that there is always something more to be done and the endless meetings, reports, audits and so on feel relentless. A challenge like climbing a mountain, with a clear start and finish-ing point, is very therapeutic for them. I've known patients who like nothing more than finishing a Lego kit to satisfy that need for completion.

Enough is a balancing act. A hobby, project or sport can become obsessive, as we touched upon in Chapter 5 (The Physical Space). Be careful what you aim for, who you compare yourself against and what you measure. If your personality is one where you must win at everything or you need it to be perfect or you can't take it or leave it, then is that activity really offering the transcen-dental space you require? When a spiritual activity starts to feel more like a burden than a release, it's probably time to re-evaluate your approach. What matters is that you have several options in this space, and you get enough opportunity to deploy them.

Accept the downside

Everything has a downside. I challenge patients who put various obstacles in their way as to why they can't do or change something to find me an example of something that doesn't have a downside. No one has come up with one yet. Maybe that suggests I'm a pessimistic person, but I like to interpret it differently. My view is everything has a downside but that shouldn't stop you from appreciating the upside. It's too easy to look at something and only see the hassle. As a result, you miss out on something that's good for you.

It's a common refrain that people will say they don't want to exercise but admit that they do feel better afterwards. It's a hassle to go to the gym or get changed into your gear and head out into the cold, wet winter nights or a baking-hot summer's day to do some exercise. Of course, there's a downside but the upside is worth it in the long run. It's easy to say no to things because you're stressed, but keeping your hexagon in order requires enough time in the spiritual space. Saying yes to a coffee with a friend or to an invitation to an event could count as an activity for your spiritual space and could be well worth the downside.

I like to think of downsides as being the price of admission. Of course there's going to be some downside but it's probably a small price to pay for the upside. If you can come to peace with that – which essentially is a spiritual outlook – then the downside feels less like a negative and more like a worthwhile price for the benefit you're getting. A few less drops in the stress bucket. And if you conclude that the upside isn't worth the downside, it may well be something that doesn't belong in your health hexagon.

My patient Orla once told me all the things she would do if she won the lottery. At the time, a large jackpot of £148 million had been won by someone in the region so it was all over the local news. I remember thinking as she reeled off all the list that she didn't need £148 million to do any of them. She was putting barriers and excuses in her way to justify not being able to do these things. She said she wanted to do things like get fit, read more books, travel. Somehow she felt she had to be a multimillionaire to create the time to do these things.

I asked her to consider whether she could do any of these things with less than £148 million. Of course she could, she said, but the barrier of time was her main justification for not doing them already. If she really wanted to do any of those (purpose), the downside would be that she needed to organise herself better.

It might involve a few sacrifices or simple changes to how she spent her days, such as perhaps reading for 20 minutes with her morning cup of coffee instead of scrolling through her phone. It's incredible how much reading you can get through in a year if you devote 20 minutes to it five days a week.

Daniel, meanwhile, told me he was going on a family holiday to San Francisco. His children were quite young, and I asked him if he thought his kids were old enough to truly get something out of it. His view was that it would never be the right time for them all to be the correct age to appreciate San Francisco. They were going so they didn't miss out and hopefully the kids would each get something from the experience. If they didn't remember it because they were too young, then so be it. This conversation, and the one with Orla, got me thinking about the things I was putting off until I had more time or more money and whether I could get on with doing some of them now.

I'd always wanted to record an album of original songs with a full band. I'd been playing and writing for years and liked the idea of making an album but never felt that I could justify doing it. It would take up time, energy and money and I thought I should wait until I had them in abundance. Maybe when I retired. Then I realised I didn't have a specific date in mind for retirement and if I took a day off now to do something unrelated to work, I could always work another day to make up for it somewhere down the line. This liberated my thinking about time.

It's too easy to think of your working life as more important than everything else and that you will get on with living after you retire. None of us know what life will look like 10 years down the line so it's important to make the most of opportunities while you have the energy and health to do so. I saw Leonard Cohen in concert in London in 2008. At the time he was 74 years old. He recalled how the last time he had played London was 15 or 16 years previously and declared that he was merely a young fella back then. Age is relative. I know 85-year-olds who wish they had the energy they had when they were 70. They think 70 is young – and so it is by comparison.

The conversations I had with my patients made me realise I was putting excuses in my own way. I decided that I would make my music project happen. The songs were written, and I had played enough on the local music scene that I knew people who could help. I blocked off a few Wednesday afternoons to go to the studio and record some guitar and vocals. I could work other Wednesdays down the line. I allowed the producer to choose the musicians to play on the album and organise sessions for them to play. I gave him the freedom to come up with the arrangements, all of which meant I didn't have to be there physically, which saved more time. He sent me edits of the various sessions, which I listened to on my runs. I reported back on the bits I liked or didn't and he tweaked them here and there. I had great fun doing the shoot for the album cover. The concept was my wife's idea. We thrashed out some thoughts over a nice meal and a few drinks one evening and her enthusiasm reassured me it was worth doing. Getting the record completed and sent off to be pressed and receiving some hard copies in the post was a nice moment. Having a launch gig where friends travelled to be there was a highlight, despite having tonsillitis on the night! Sending it out into the world on all the usual digital platforms was another milestone.

The best part for me though was listening to those raw edits on my runs. For me, that was spiritual. It was this album, these pieces of music that I had written, coming to life and only the producer and I at that point had ever heard them. As I ran past traffic or through a park or along a river where others walked and talked and ran on cold wet November nights, I had a warm fuzzy feeling; this tiny piece of something unique that mattered to me at a deep level and only I was experiencing it at that moment. It's a strange kind of freedom. Others might get the same feeling from jumping out of an aeroplane.

Getting that balance right where a project fulfils a spiritual need without drifting into work or becoming a burden can be a challenge. I've seen plenty of patients start something for the purpose of their spiritual space only for it to turn into another thing they must succeed at or put pressure on themselves to be good enough. They are missing the point. You don't have to measure everything. You don't have to be brilliant at everything. What you need is something you can get lost in.

People have asked me why I don't make more of an effort to sell and promote the album. For me, that project was about getting an album done. It was nothing to do with making a career in music or an expectation that it would be listened to. It's out there and it's nice to see that it has been played in over 40 countries through different streaming platforms. It's amazing to think that maybe someone in the Philippines, United States, Mexico or Georgia is listening to a song of mine while out for their run too and maybe it's helping their health hexagon. I didn't need to win the lottery to make it happen. I didn't need to be retired. I didn't need to turn it into a job. I didn't need to live up to the expectations of others. I didn't need to compete against other songwriters for it to give me what I needed from it. Yes, I had to be organised. Yes, I had to devote some energy to it. Yes, it did have its ups and downs along the way, but that's the price of admission.

Life is an 80 per cent game

In 1906 Vilfredo Pareto noticed that 80 per cent of the wealth in Italy was owned by 20 per cent of the population. This 80/20 ratio occurred again and again, even in his garden where 20 per cent of the pods contained 80 per cent of the peas. The 80/20 rule or Pareto principle pops up all over the place. Companies have identified that 80 per cent of the complaints come from 20 per cent of the customers. Apparently 20 per cent of activities will account for 80 per cent of the value of what you do. It's even found in the mass of the planets of our solar system with 20 per cent of the planets making up 80 per cent of the total mass.[11]

It's easy to make statistics say whatever you want them to, but the 80/20 ratio is a useful guiding principle to managing life in the modern world. It can be really helpful to leave yourself a bit of space so you have a margin for error and capacity to deal with the unexpected. If your diary is only ever 80 per cent full, you can manage the inevitable delays, niggles and frustrations that are part of everyday living without getting flustered. You have factored in space for the known unknowns.

Consider your best average day. What does it look like? For me it means I'm up and showered on time. I make a coffee for my wife, and I get to read for 20 minutes in peace as I have breakfast before the kids get up. The kids have breakfast, I read with the youngest and they both do their spelling homework or times tables before we cycle to school. They get in on time and I get to work promptly. My appointments all run smoothly and to time. Some appointments force me to think and challenge myself, but not all of them. I have time for a coffee and something to eat and time to go to the toilet when necessary.

I'll get my clinical notes done and leave on time. If it's a running day I get into my gear, put a podcast on and do 5 km, finishing at my youngest son's after-school club. We'll get in, have a healthy snack, do homework and music practice without arguments or resistance. My wife will arrive home from a good day at work and maybe go for a run with the older one so they have some time together. We have dinner together where we chat about our day and hopefully have a laugh as well as get the boys thinking about something that challenges them. My wife will put the younger one to bed, so she has some one-to-one time with him too. Then she and I have a couple of hours to relax together in front of the fire and watch some TV. That's my best average day. No surprises, no delays, everyone fed, happy, exercised, challenged but not overwhelmed.

If you push yourself to the limit every day, you set the bar higher and higher and sooner or later the minimum is not sustainable. That absolutely doesn't mean you coast along and never push yourself, but consider how sustainable your expectations of what you can do on an average day are. If you're pushing yourself to achieve more and more in a day, you start to believe that it's possible to do that every day. Your health hexagon is likely to disagree.

When I worked at the London Olympics in 2012, I remember watching Bradley Wiggins winning a gold medal in the time trial. He became the first man in history to win the Tour de France and an Olympic gold medal in the same year. In fact, it was the same month. We often think of Olympians needing to be at the peak of their powers to win. Wiggins didn't peak for either event, but he did prime for both of them. If you peak there is only one direction you can go in and that's down, but if you prime that's something you can sustain.

I have no idea if Wiggins's average speed or wattage or whatever other metric you could consider adhered to the Pareto principle, but I think it's a valuable tool when considering how you go about your day and the challenges you set for yourself. Your best average day is where you prime, not peak. There will be days when you need to be at your peak, but that can't be your default. It's not sustainable. Remember, if you are living in an unsustainable way, that is pro-inflammatory and your pain system will speak up to grab your attention.

Creative time

Time is usually the barrier or excuse to avoid the spiritual space. This space is not just about switching off, getting lost or recalibrating to your true self. It's also about opportunities to think differently, which might just prove to make you more productive or successful in other parts of your hexagon. If you set preschool children a creative task – such as how many ways can you think of to use a paper clip? – the vast majority of them will come up with a huge number of different ideas. Adults will come up with perhaps 10 or 15. Children at this age are not confined by the rules of society or blinkered by experience or limited by the threat of failure. They are inventive, creative and fearless. They might suggest using a paper clip as a big neon slide or making a cake the shape of a paper clip.

As we get older, we are far less likely to adopt unfamiliar hypotheses; instead we resort to the existing bank of knowledge we have gathered to come up with a solution to a problem even though this may be less consistent with the evidence available. We are less likely to explore new ways of creative problem-solving in the way that children or teenagers might take risks and try out new ideas.

It is now generally accepted that diversity of thinking and creativity help push boundaries, allow for cross-pollination of ideas between industries and offer novel solutions to problems. A study comparing Nobel Prize-winning scientists with other scientists from the same era discovered that the Nobel Laureates were twice as likely to play a musical instrument, seven times more likely to draw, paint or sculpt, twelve times more likely to write poetry, plays or popular books, and twenty-two times as likely to perform at amateur acting, dancing or magic.[12]

It is time to look at the spiritual space differently: rather than see it as a waste of time or indulgence, see it as an essential use of time. Spending time in places and situations that challenge you to think differently can help get you out of a fixed way of thinking and spark solutions to problems. This is as true for pain as it is for anything else in life. You can only filter your pain experience based on the information you have. To change this, you have to try looking at things a little differently and broaden your bank of information to draw on when negotiating with the elements that contribute to the pain experience. The spiritual space can help you switch off and get lost but it can also help you find something. Spend some time doing something different, something creative until you discover what's enough for you. It might be a much more efficient use of your time.

Worry time

It is possible to negotiate with your pain system. It's also possible to negotiate with your worries. A psychologist I treated once told me how she suggested to patients who worried a lot to put aside 15 minutes a day of worry time. Life goes on around you and no matter what you are worrying about, you still have to deal with the day-to-day tasks of life. She advised her patients that if they found worries popping into their head during the day, rather than letting them sit in the background while they tried to get on with whatever they were doing, they should acknowledge the worry and say, "I'll deal with you in my worry time." During that worry time they would talk and think about their problem and how it should be managed that day or the next day. Outside of that worry time they were not to think about it or talk about it. They had to consciously tell themselves to stop. Of course, this didn't mean that their worries had been magically resolved; what it meant was that they were in control, not their worries.

The more time you spend worrying the more energy it takes, and you need to get through your day, which requires energy too. As always with the health hexagon, you need a direction of travel. A coach once told me that a problem without a plan is like a glass of milk left out of the fridge. If you don't move it, it will curdle. The simplest thing you can do is have a plan to deal with worries popping into your head. The plan is scheduled worry time. That way you acknowledge it but schedule time to address it rather than allowing it to dominate your life. The psychologist who explained this to me also said, "It's very hard to worry about something for a solid 15 minutes when you concentrate on it, but you can let it worry you all day if you're not careful."

Another patient I was dealing with told me that he played golf to relax and get away from the stresses of work. He was a reasonably good golfer, but he didn't worry too much about how he played. For him it was about getting out on the course and away from the office. I asked him if he ever noticed that other golfers he played with who had retired no longer had any of that work stress. How they looked like they no longer carried that weight of work on them. He agreed but then said, "Have you ever noticed how much they worry about their golf?" It got us talking about the fact that we always have space in our life for worry. I suspect most of us can find something to worry about even when everything looks like it's going fine. Maybe it's part of the human condition. If so, it's worth keeping them in perspective and not letting those worries take over.

I regularly see middle-aged patients with a painful knee or hip who are distressed that this represents the beginning of the end. Pain is a threat to your well-being. It challenges your sense of self and trust in your body. It's easy to catastrophise and before long that worry becomes all-consuming or gets blown out of proportion. It's not uncommon for patients in that situation to declare in some distress, "I just don't want to get old." Depending on the circumstances my response is something like, "Oh, but you do. Consider the alternative. If you're not getting older that means you're already dead." This usually allows them to accept that they don't want the alternative, but they are worried about getting older and what that might look like. My job as a physio is to help them get a sense of perspective and a direction of travel. A plan to improve the situation. This doesn't by any means dismiss the anxiety they might be experiencing, but if you get stuck in catastrophising you go nowhere – or worse, fall into chaos.

Chaos in this situation means feeling like you are out of control. Order is regaining a sense of perspective, considering your options, getting help from people who can give you a plan and a direction of travel. People who have travelled that road before and can help you see there is a lot of good living in front of you. This doesn't always mean you can continue with the same life you had. If you have severe knee arthritis, your marathon-running and squash-playing days are behind you. You will have to come to peace with that, but it doesn't mean you can't reorganise your health hexagon to find purpose, fulfilment and contentment.

Throughout life we move on from one phase to another. Maybe your squash days are over, but you could do an alternative sport. You can still spend enough time in the physical space and get the fulfilment you need from it in terms of exercise and camaraderie and competition, but catastrophising or refusing to accept that this phase has ended and find an alternative isn't going to help.

When you get injured or experience pain, chances are you will go through the stages of grief. It happens with every injury but the speed at which you go through these phases varies, as does the order and overall duration. Some people get stuck in a particular phase and some will go through one more than once.

If I do something as simple as bang my elbow on the frame of a door as I walk through it, I will go through the various stages just as much as if I break my leg or do something more serious. Initially it's denial. I can't believe I've whacked my elbow. I was just walking through a door. Then it's anger. At the door, at the reason I had to walk through the door. Anger at myself. Then there's guilt or bargaining depending on the severity of the injury. Guilt because my painful elbow might mean I can't work and I'm letting my patients down or I won't be able to do some DIY job I'd promised to get done. Bargaining if it's something more serious. If only the traffic lights weren't green. If only I went a different route. If only I made a different decision. Then it's depression. Why me? The inflammatory process starts and contributes to these feelings.*

---

* As part of your defence system, you have cells called macrophages. Consider these like soldiers defending your tissues and organs. They cover the lining of your

Eventually there's acceptance. You've whacked your elbow. It's sore but it's happened before and it's not the end of the world. It'll be bruised perhaps and tender for a few days but it's OK. If you have some experience of banging your elbow, you'll probably reach acceptance quicker as you have some frame of reference, which is

skin, gut, blood vessels, eyes and more, ready to defend against threat. When the body is under some form of threat, such as invading bacteria or a cut or injury, the macrophages go to work to attack that threat. They try to kill that bacteria or eat away at the injured tissue to stimulate fresh growth of new tissue. Macrophages produce by-products called cytokines and release these into the bloodstream. In part these cytokines act as a signalling system to alert macrophages in other areas of the body that they are needed elsewhere. The macrophages then get mobilised to the injured area, bringing about some of the clinical features of inflammation, such as a hot, red and swollen area. The body does a lot of its repair at night-time so you will get an increase in blood flow to the injured area at night and therefore more inflammation. This is why things are often more painful at night, which can make it difficult to sleep. However, there is another reason for that too.

In his excellent book *The Inflamed Mind: A Radical New Approach to Depression*, psychiatrist Professor Edward Bullmore explains why we can feel depressed when we are inflamed. The cytokines enter the brain and this influences the balance of mood-stabilising chemicals such as serotonin. He suggests that getting depressed while injured is an important preservation mechanism. Think of it this way. Back in the days of hunter-gatherers, why would it be an advantage to feel miserable when you had cut yourself on a branch out hunting? Why would it help to avoid others, which depressed people tend to do? The biggest risk for you back then was infection. If you isolated yourself from the group, you reduced your risk of infection. People often feel uncomfortable around people who are depressed so they isolate themselves from you too, broadening that safety cordon.

Features of depression also include remorse and pessimism, which could be a way of helping you learn from your mistakes and avoid them in future. You may lose your appetite, which means you are not taking resources from the group. Poor sleep is also a feature of depression, which means you can stay alert to additional threats from predators while you are injured. Effectively acting as night watch for the group and alerting them to danger means you make yourself useful and are more likely to be welcomed back into the group as you recover. All of this could improve your chances of survival.

Tens of thousands if not millions of years of evolution led to such a mechanism. Today we have better medical care, antibiotics and systems to take care of the sick and vulnerable, but it takes tens of thousands of years to breed out such genes, so we are likely to continue to feel somewhat miserable when we get inflamed.

very important (see Chapter 11, Stored Data). If you don't have some prior experience, you might get stuck in denial or anger.

Let yourself be happy

Number five on Bronnie Ware's list of regrets is "I wish I had let myself be happier." This was surprisingly common, she explains: "Many did not realise until the end that happiness is a choice. They had stayed stuck in old patterns and habits. The so-called 'comfort' of familiarity overflowed into their emotions, as well as their physical lives. Fear of change had them pretending to others, and to their selves, that they were content, when deep within, they longed to laugh properly and have silliness in their life again."[13]

My patient Neil was given a friend's apartment in New York for a summer. No fees, just the keys. He went for a couple of months. On his return I asked what he did in New York. He told me he never moved more than a couple of blocks from the apartment the entire time he was there. Time just kind of slipped away. He kept thinking he would do all these wonderful things and he had loads of time, so he didn't feel any urgency to get on with it. Before he knew it, he had wasted the chance. He also said he felt a bit guilty about doing fun things when other people in his life were working or not there to enjoy them and that it seemed somehow a bit easier not to do them.

Don't hide your happiness. Recognise an opportunity when it presents itself because it may never happen again.

After graduating I went travelling. I stopped off in Fiji for a couple of weeks. White sandy beaches, palm trees tilting towards the shore, bath-temperature water, lush mountainous terrain, flying fish, spectacular underwater caves, beautiful coral, no light pollution. When it's a cloudless night you can lie back on a beach, listening to the gentle sound of waves lapping up around you and see millions of stars. The sky becomes more white than black as you gaze upon the vastness of the universe. It's my idea of paradise.

While I was there, I got chatting to a local girl on one of Fiji's 300 islands. She was miserable, she said. I was young so didn't have the insight I have now, but I couldn't believe that anyone could be miserable there. Why was she sad? I asked. She looked onto the horizon and said. "I'll never get off this place." At first I couldn't understand, but then it was obvious. Paradise wasn't this for her. Big concrete buildings, flashing neon signs, traffic, noise, excitement, the chaos of a big urban sprawl was what she wanted.

She was frustrated that all these backpackers were coming to her island and telling her stories of the big cities they came from. She would never see these places or was very unlikely to. All these privileged backpackers, of which I was one, made her feel more and more miserable with every tale of how wonderful somewhere else was. I tried to explain as best I could that we came there because we thought what she had was paradise, but I don't know if that made things better or worse.

It helped me understand that no matter where I am, it's paradise to someone somewhere and that reminding myself of that helps me to embrace it and to be grateful. It's great to get away and experience new things and different places, if you are fortunate enough to be able to, but it's just as good to embrace where you are. The grass can seem greener elsewhere for sure, but if bombs aren't falling on your head, where you are maybe isn't so bad.

I always think the hospital is full of people who'd love to be doing what I'm doing now. That's not to say that everyone is in a great place. We can all pontificate about what we would do if this or that happened, but the reality is no one knows for

129

certain. I don't know how I'd respond to being paralysed or given a particular diagnosis. What I'm saying is, appreciate what it is you do have.

Carrots are good for you

You'll have figured out by now that one of the main points of getting your health hexagon in order is having a direction of travel. In the spiritual space this can be having something to look forward to, something to act as a carrot dangling as a reward for managing the downsides that come with life. For me that might be a gig or a play or a day date with my wife. It's easier for us to take some time off work and go for lunch or a walk and a catch-up while the kids are at school rather than trying to find a babysitter and then deal with busy pubs and restaurants. I've personally found that if there's less dependency on other moving parts for the spiritual activities of your health hexagon, you're more likely to be successful in doing the thing you need. If you've arranged things so you can take a day off here and there, then chances are you are not doing so bad at getting your hexagon in order. That's a feat worth acknowledging in itself.

If you discover that you need something in your life then book the time off well in advance and commit to it. Negotiate with those around you to make it happen. If you need a night out with your old school friends because it's likely to mean you laugh so hard you can't breathe for a moment, explain why that's important for you and what you can offer in return. Perhaps your partner is only too happy for you to have a night like that every now and again because they want to watch a TV programme they never otherwise get a chance to, or they want some time for themselves somewhere else down the line. If those around you can see how these things make you a better person to be around, they'll want you to do those things too. Enough can be win-win for everyone.

Over the years patients have told me all sorts of wonderful things they do which fall into the spiritual space. The occasional visit to the seaside, a weekend in the mountains annually, a couple of days at a festival drinking warm beer and eating bad chips, or a walk in a forest. Window-shopping, people-watching, jigsaws, colouring-in books, watching bubble-gum TV, learning Arabic, sanding a piece of wood. A nursery worker by day, a fierce wrestling persona on Tuesday nights. A villain in a play, a dame in a pantomime, a mime artist, a football fan.

The spiritual space gives you permission to be. To take a break from the pressures of other areas of your life. To fill you with energy, to inspire, to play, to drop the masks or wear a different one. To tune in to the world around you or tune out of the world you're in. It gives you a reason to be, and a connection to things bigger than yourself. To accept the passage of time, to look forward, to gain perspective, to be grateful, to bring order to chaos or chaos to order. To help counterbalance a world that contributes to a pro-inflammatory life and reduce the sensitivity of your stress response system. To give you moments of peace, moments of calm, moments of tranquillity.

Now, let's go to sleep.

CHAPTER 9

Sleep

GIVEN WE SPEND a third of our life asleep and we would die without it, sleep is clearly an essential part of survival, but the way we live today doesn't always facilitate a healthy relationship with sleep. By the end of this chapter, having looked at the impact sleep has on your memory, immune system, inflammation, mood and stress systems, as well as the impact exercise has on sleep and diet, I hope you will value sleep just as much as the other parts of your health hexagon and be ready to work towards getting enough sleep for you.

The basics

Circadian rhythms are physical, mental and behavioural changes that follow a 24-hour cycle. It is actually thought to be 24 hours and 11 minutes plus or minus 16 minutes rather than precisely 24 hours, so arguably living to a 24-hour clock already involves trying to force your body into an "unnatural pattern".[1] This "body clock" responds to and is calibrated by exposure to light and dark. Your body clock "pacemaker", the suprachiasmatic nucleus (SCN) in the hypothalamus, is synchronised by sunlight entering your retinas.[2] For those in the West, particularly in northern European countries, the winter months offer relatively limited exposure to daylight. We live in centrally heated houses and work in sealed office buildings. Although you might sit by a window, modern glass filters UV light and therefore exposure to direct sunlight is limited. Artificial lighting, particularly from screens during the evening, makes synchronising your natural body clock even more challenging.

Not everyone has the same sleep pattern. Roughly speaking, 40 per cent of people are early birds; 30 per cent are night owls; and the remaining 30 per cent are something in between, but lean slightly towards the evening type. Research varies on the exact percentages of people who fall into each category but your chronotype – the pattern you follow most closely – is strongly determined by your genetic make-up.[3]

Having different sleep patterns is probably helpful from a tribal standpoint, enabling different members of a group to provide function and security at different hours of the day. Teenagers across the globe tend to become night owls and sleep longer into the late morning or early afternoon. In part this allows the next generation to separate themselves from their parents by living to different schedules and allowing for a little independence. As teenage brains go through a remarkable rate of growth, development and reorganisation, longer sleep periods are also important for memory and emotional stability.[4] Once through those teenage years, the chronotype usually emerges.

Your chronotype will affect your productivity. A morning person will be most productive early in the day while an evening person will struggle to be on top form for an early morning meeting. As with everything, figuring out enough for you is important. If you are a night owl who struggles to get to sleep before midnight, no matter how hard you try to force yourself into an early bird's schedule by getting up at 6 a.m., you may end up missing on average two hours of sleep a night. This will have a significant impact on your memory as your brain processes and consolidates the activities of the day into your memory bank as you sleep. The figure that keeps coming up in the research is 40 per cent less consolidation of memory than you should have on account of poor sleep.[5]

It seems a ludicrous waste of your time to work hard during the day only to undo that work by not getting enough sleep. Information is temporarily stored in the hippocampus as short-term memory and then filed away into long-term memory when you sleep. If you don't sleep well on Tuesday night, you won't remember as much of Tuesday. Many people report that they can function perfectly well on only three to four hours' sleep a night, but frankly the evidence doesn't seem to support this. You might be able to do it, but it doesn't mean that there isn't a price to pay.

There are two types of sleep: rapid eye movement or REM sleep and non-rapid eye movement or NREM sleep. In a normal sleep cycle, you go from NREM to REM sleep every 90 minutes, but the amount of time spent in NREM or REM varies across cycles. NREM sleep is further divided into light NREM and deep NREM sleep. All three phases are essential. Deep NREM sleep occurs early in the sleep cycle and is important for fact-based learning. You can influence what memories are saved by consciously asking your brain to remember before you fall asleep. When I write a new song, I sing it to myself as I'm falling asleep. It's amazing how well I can remember the lyrics by doing this. I might not play that song again for weeks or months but it's in there on automatic pilot. Motor memory, such as the mechanics of playing sport or musical instruments, is consolidated by type 2 NREM sleep, which happens more in the last two hours of an eight-hour sleep cycle. As you go through various phases of NREM and REM every 90 minutes it's not exclusive to that window, but getting six hours rather than eight will have an impact on memory and performance.

REM sleep, typically the dream phase of sleep, is also important for processing emotions experienced that day.* Alcohol suppresses REM sleep, which can account for poorer memory of events on a night involving alcohol. If you want a drink with your meal, there is an argument for having a glass of wine with lunch rather than dinner, so that the alcohol has been processed before you go to bed. However, the risk is the drinking continues as a result of an early start!

The amount of time you give yourself to be available for sleep is very important. Your chronotype means you might get to bed early, but it doesn't mean you fall asleep as soon as you go to bed. It does however mean that if you don't get to bed, you're unlikely to get to sleep – unless of course you fall asleep on the sofa before you go to bed. This has consequences too.

When we are awake, we produce a chemical called adenosine. This builds up the longer we are awake and produces what is known as sleep pressure. Think of that as tiredness. Melatonin

---

* It does this in the absence of norepinephrine, which allows you to process the memory without stress and anxiety; see Claude Gottesmann, "The Involvement of Noradrenaline in Rapid Eye Movement Sleep Mentation", *Frontiers in Neurology* 2 (12 December 2011): 81, https://doi.org/10.3389/fneur.2011.00081. This will be important when we take a look at pain memory. It is thought that this mechanism may play a role in developing post-traumatic stress disorder (PTSD) as norepinephrine levels are higher in those who have PTSD and norepinephrine is known to disrupt REM sleep; see Edward F. Pace-Schott, Anne Germain, and Mohammed R. Milad, "Sleep and REM Sleep Disturbance in the Pathophysiology of PTSD: The Role of Extinction Memory", *Biology of Mood & Anxiety Disorders* 5 (29 May 2015): 3. https://doi.org/10.1186/s13587-015-0018-9.

is a natural hormone your body produces in line with darkness, signalling to your circadian rhythm that it's time for sleep. The combination of these three things (adenosine, melatonin/darkness, circadian rhythm) helps us fall asleep. As we get older, changes to our circadian rhythm and melatonin levels make us want to fall asleep earlier, so it's not uncommon to drift off to sleep before it's time for bed. The problem with that is falling asleep washes out your adenosine so when you do wake up and head for bed, you won't have the sleep pressure to help you fall asleep. This can make you think you're an insomniac. Wearing sunglasses in the morning and getting daylight exposure in the afternoon can help calibrate your circadian rhythm so you are less likely to fall asleep on the sofa before bed.

Caffeine blocks adenosine receptors, making you feel more awake. The half-life of caffeine is five to seven hours, meaning a cup at noon is still 50 per cent potent at 7 p.m. When caffeine is finally processed by a liver enzyme, all the stored adenosine floods the receptors and creates a caffeine crash. Some people process caffeine quicker than others, which is why some people seem able to have a double espresso shortly before bedtime without any ill effect. They are a rare species.

Artificial light can disrupt your sleep, particularly during the evening. Research looking at short wavelength light from 90 minutes of smart phone use before bed suggests that it affects night-time alertness, melatonin levels, circadian rhythm and drowsiness the next day. These effects were only marginally reduced by a light filter.[6] A meta-analysis of 467 studies involving 125,198 children between 6 and 19 years old showed strong and consistent association between bedtime media device use and inadequate sleep quantity, poor sleep quality and excessive daytime sleepiness.[7] Shifting your sleep cycle by just an hour as happens with daylight saving time when clocks go forward especially in the spring has been associated with a modest rise in heart attack symptoms in the week following the clock change. As a result the European Parliament are considering abolishing daylight saving time and are carrying out more in-depth analysis of the health implications.[8]

The amount of time you give yourself in bed, the amount of daylight and artificial light exposure you have, when and how much alcohol and caffeine you consume all influence how well you sleep and consequently how well your memory functions. If you value your memory and this is a strong enough purpose for you, then you won't spend hours on devices before bedtime. Why not read a book instead? You might say that you can't avoid working on the laptop in the evening as work is so busy, but that just tells me you are burying yourself in the mental space at the expense of other parts of your hexagon. Is it worth it? Maybe the impact poor sleep has on other metrics of well-being will help you re-evaluate its importance.

Cortisol and stress

The stress hormone cortisol is an important component of the HPA axis (see Chapter 7). It contributes to energy distribution and is pivotal to your sleep-wake cycle. Cortisol has its own circadian rhythm to help meet your genetic sleep requirements. When processed at the right times and the right amount, cortisol helps you wake up in the morning and fall asleep and stay asleep in the night. In the morning, light stimulates the suprachiasmatic nucleus, letting your body know to release cortisol, norepinephrine and serotonin to wake you up and keep you alert.[9] That early-morning surge of cortisol (the cortisol awakening response or CAR) gives you an energy boost and lasts for 30–45 minutes, returning to baseline after about an hour.[10] It's thought that this CAR process is very sensitive to heat: your body temperature increases by approximately 1 degree C in the morning to trigger these hormonal signals.[11] This might help to explain why it's often harder to wake up in the dark, cold winter months.

As the day goes on, your cortisol levels decline, reaching their lowest around midnight. About two to three hours after you fall asleep cortisol production increases again, rising to help wake you up in the morning. If you are a night owl your cortisol cycle will be later, meaning you are more sluggish and less alert than your early-bird counterparts. Sleeping past your usual rising time diminishes your CAR and leads to that sleep hangover feeling.

Cortisol is also important in the storage of memory, especially emotionally negative memories. There is an abundance of cortisol receptors in the amygdala (the threat detector part of your brain) and hippocampus (responsible for memory processing). When it comes to memory, the brain filters experiences that happen during the day and prioritises those that are emotionally salient.[12] We are designed to remember strongly negative emotions or experiences over neutral ones to help protect us for the future. Cortisol plays a role here: elevated cortisol levels at night have been shown to improve memory storage.[13,14] For example, let's say you're walking down the street and a dog in a garden barks at you aggressively and runs to the gate, giving you a bit of a shock. Your HPA axis kicks into gear and produces cortisol; you might jump or run out of the way. Your heart is pounding from adrenaline. You might feel a little anxious for a few hours.

That night as you sleep, elevated cortisol levels will process that event. If that processing is done properly in the absence of norepinephrine, you will take some of the anxiety out of the experience. You will remember there is an aggressive dog at that particular house, but you won't be terrified to walk past. Your memory will help you prepare for and deal with a similar situation in the future. It has also been shown that if cortisol levels are too high during waking hours, this interferes with your ability to retrieve information.[15] Excessive cortisol has been shown to cause atrophy or shrinkage of the hippocampus, which can have a significant impact on memory.[16] Enough is key. Enough cortisol to help you remember; not so much that it causes you to forget.

The body has three nervous systems: the central nervous system, which is the brain and spinal cord; the peripheral nervous system (the nerves coming off the central nervous system to provide sensation and power); and the autonomic nervous system or ANS. The ANS is divided into two opposing systems: the sympathetic nervous system (SNS), which is the "fight-or-flight" response, and the parasympathetic nervous system (PNS), which is the "rest-and-digest" response. The HPA axis influences the balance of the ANS to prioritise resources if there's a threat. In a threat situation, perceived or otherwise, your HPA axis is activated. You produce cortisol, your PNS is dialled down and your SNS is dialled up to produce the hormone epinephrine (adrenaline) and the neurotransmitter norepinephrine. This keeps you alert and increases your heart rate. In normal circumstances a short-lived stress will eventually switch off the HPA axis as cortisol levels rise and the PNS will dial back up to restore balance.

This is all well and good if the stress is brief. If, however, you are living in a stressful environment with work pressures, family difficulties, financial woes, one thing after another, then you will be constantly producing cortisol and your HPA axis will be continuously stimulated. Your SNS will keep producing epinephrine and norepinephrine, giving you a faster resting heart rate and increased core body temperature. That makes it more difficult to fall asleep and your sleep cycle will suffer. Elevated cortisol levels make it harder to move from lighter to deeper sleep cycles, and the combination of norepinephrine and cortisol could contribute to higher levels of anxiety when it comes to processing emotionally salient events. This all leads to sleep debt, tiredness, poor memory recall and difficulty concentrating. All further contributing to generating stress.

In the right proportions, cortisol acts as an anti-inflammatory, but if you're sleep-deprived, the cortisol response can become dysfunctional. Rather than reducing inflammation, it can become pro-inflammatory. Shift workers whose sleep patterns work against their natural body clock have been shown to have higher levels of inflammation, which leads to chronic disease. Excess cortisol can cause high blood pressure, type 2 diabetes and obesity[17] and there is also an association between chronic stress, cortisol levels, loss of libido and erectile dysfunction.[18]

As sleep is an important part of cortisol's circadian rhythm, even a few hours of sleep loss can result in higher concentrations of cortisol the next night. That makes it harder to fall asleep[19] and you end up with a vicious cycle of finding it harder and harder to get quality sleep. The good news is that reducing cortisol levels can reverse the changes to the hippocampus.[20]

If the threat to your memory, the risk of heart disease and

diabetes or sexual dysfunction weren't good enough reasons to prioritise sleep, maybe the impact sleep has on your immune system will seal the deal.

Immune and inflammatory considerations

Sleep is when the body repairs and prepares. Muscles, injuries and wounds repair during sleep, which is why professional athletes try to ensure they have eight hours a night and often take naps after training sessions in the day. Waste products are removed as you sleep, and the immune system prepares itself to protect you from illness and infection for the following day. It's also been shown that sleep helps with the antibody response to vaccination.[21] A study in 2002 showed that sleep significantly impacts your response to a standard flu vaccine. Those who had between seven and nine hours of sleep in the week before getting the vaccine generated a stronger antibody reaction than those who had their sleep restricted to four hours a night in the week preceding their vaccine. The sleep-deprived group produced less than 50 per cent of the immune response of the rested group. Even when allowed two to three weeks of recovery sleep to get over the week of sleep deprivation, they didn't develop a full immune reaction to the flu vaccine.[22] Similar results are seen with hepatitis A and B vaccines.[23]

Broadly speaking, your immune system can be divided into two categories: innate immunity, which is a multisystem generalised defence; and adaptive immunity, which is what you develop and becomes more targeted to a specific threat. One of the first lines of defence is leukocytes or white blood cells. When they detect a foreign pathogen (an organism that can cause disease) they release cytokines to signal an attack is happening and that can alert macrophages, which we came across in the inflammatory response (see *The Inflamed Mind* footnote on page 126 in Chapter 8). The innate immune system signals that there is an attack by a foreign substance. The adaptive immune response can learn to deal with the specific attack and therefore mount a more sophisticated defence when it comes across that pathogen in the future – for example, developing specific antibodies to a common cold. The immune system has to keep a fine balance between being strong enough to find and defend against potential threats but also not overreacting and attacking unnecessarily. Sleep has been shown to play a role in keeping this delicate balance.[24]

Certain things will trigger stronger reactions in some people than others. If you suffer from hay fever you will know this already. A certain pollen can trigger an aggressive histamine response in some people and not others. If your defence system sees that pollen as a dangerous pathogen, it will go to work, causing streaming, itching eyes, a runny nose and a headache. The same pollen generates no reaction from someone else.

Sleep and the immune system are intertwined, and a lack of sleep can make the immune system less capable of defending but also overreact. Someone once described it to me like a bouncer at a nightclub. If the bouncer is assessing risk reasonably, when they see someone bump into another person and spill a drink they might observe from afar. They will look to see if the person who caused the spill did so accidentally, if they apologise and if everyone seems happy. If so, they let it go. But if that bouncer is feeling particularly vigilant because he's having a bad day or has been drinking double espressos for four hours and he is supercharged and irritable, he might well react aggressively, dragging that clumsy individual out. Their friends protest and before too long you have a volatile situation. A stimulated HPA axis and stressed immune system due to lack of sleep effectively behave the same way.

During sleep, certain elements of the immune system become more active. Your body is trying to repair itself, which is why injuries are often more painful at night-time: you get an increase in blood flow to the injured part, causing swelling, heat and tenderness. It's usually a good sign if you can sleep on the injured part and sleep through the night. Typically, this suggests it's no longer actively inflamed.

Your ability to fight infection also suffers due to lack of sleep. T cells are a type of white blood cell that alerts the body to a pathogen (helper T cells) and attacks it (cytotoxic T cells). Studies comparing those who get a full eight hours' sleep versus those who stay awake all night have shown that T cells' ability to bind to infected cells or other immune cells is diminished.[25] Natural killer (NK) cells destroy cells taken over by pathogens. Reducing sleep to four hours a night, even for one night, has shown a reduction in NK cells by 72 per cent.[26] Restricting sleep to six hours a night has been shown to increase your risk of getting the common cold by as much as 4.2 times.[27] There is a two-way relationship between sleep and the immune system:[28] when you are fighting an illness, you will often sleep longer so your immune system can work more effectively.

If all of that wasn't enough, poor sleep can also make you sore. A bad night's sleep can leave you 42 per cent more sensitive to thermal pain stimulus.[29] Inflammatory markers sensitise the pain system by making nociceptive fibres more sensitive (see Chapter 3, The Sensory Bus Ride).[30] People with persistent pain frequently sleep poorly and have raised inflammatory markers.[31]

Mental health

We can all feel cranky after a bad night's sleep. The US public health agency the Centers for Disease Control and Prevention reports that one-third of adults in the US get less than the recommended eight hours of sleep a night.[32] In the short term you will feel tired and irritable, and beyond the physical consequences, you are more likely to worsen depression. Sleep and mental health are closely intertwined. Many mental health conditions are associated with problematic sleeping; poor sleep can also exacerbate mental health problems.[33,34] Conversely this could also suggest that interventions designed to improve sleep could help your mental health.

Acute sleep deprivation can cause feelings of anxiety and depression specifically, and general distress more broadly, in physically and psychologically healthy adults.[35] Even short periods of sleep deprivation can increase levels of anxiety. Sustained sleep loss can have a causal effect. Sleep difficulties are also seen in PTSD, bipolar disorder and ADHD, with some studies showing improvements in the severity of ADHD symptoms with sleep interventions.[36] Improving sleep isn't a cure for such conditions but it can help reduce their severity, while the research suggests that improving sleep may reduce the risk of developing some mental health problems. A 2021 study in the *Journal of American Medical Association Psychiatry* looked at 840,000 adults, some of whom had experienced major depressive episodes, and showed that going to sleep an hour earlier reduced the risk of a major depressive episode by 23 per cent.[37]

So the evidence is strong that sleep deprivation has significant consequences for your physical and mental health. What can you do about it? The single most important factor when it comes to sleep is getting enough time in bed to sleep. If you don't give yourself the chance to get eight hours, how do you expect to get eight hours? It comes down to purpose again. If you believe that you need sleep, then you can set the conditions to help you sleep. This means organising your day to facilitate it. You'll want some daylight exposure to help calibrate your circadian rhythm daily. You might double this up with your exercise routine so that you can have your run, walk or cycle in the sunshine. You'll regulate your caffeine and alcohol intake and reduce your exposure to screens in the evening. This will require discipline and trust in your own abilities. Work demands are often the greatest threat to your ability to give yourself sleep opportunity – email in particular.

Large organisations such as water companies use the term "leakage" when making decisions that support or interfere with their purpose. It will cost them too much time, energy and money to fix all the leaking water pipes, so they just accept that there will be some leakage in the system, as long as it doesn't stop them providing their core service. Are there areas in your life where you can adopt the same philosophy rather than wasting hours on trying to obtain perfection? This could just allow you to get into your comfortable bed on time for a good night's sleep. More refreshed the next morning, better concentration, better memory recall, less irritable, healthier, less stressed and less and less leakage as a result.

Now, what about the bed itself?

Seven mattresses

As a physio I regularly get asked to identify the "best" pillow or mattress. I also regularly hear from patients that they have hurt their back or neck because they "slept wrong" and want to know what the best position to sleep in is. It won't surprise you to hear that my philosophy on this is that you should do what feels right for you. There isn't any robust evidence out there to say that one mattress is scientifically better for you than another when it comes to normal domestic use. (Don't be misled by the word "orthopaedic" when it comes to describing a mattress; it's not a protected title.) Studies have suggested that the average preference for mattress firmness is medium-firm.[38] Preference is subjective, but it's somewhere to start from.

Studies looking at pillow materials, shapes and height haven't identified an optimum set-up. An analysis of 167 articles published since 1997 on the ergonomic considerations of pillows reviewed the research and concluded that "achieving optimal cervical spine alignment, appropriate pressure distribution, and minimal muscle activity during sleep cannot yet be identified considering the lack of sufficient evidence. Moreover, there remain no firm conclusions about the optimal pillow height for the supine and lateral positions."[39] My view is that if your body is asleep, it's happy. Don't stress about the right pillow or mattress. If it helps to have a specific pillow and it allows you to sleep better, by all means include it in your hexagon. I definitely like my pillow, but I don't bring it on holiday with me.

You've chosen a mattress and a pillow. What about the best position to sleep in? There is no right or wrong position. If you're asleep, you're happy. Let me qualify that. If you sleep naturally, you're happy. It's not unheard of for people under the influence of drugs or alcohol or following a head injury to fall asleep in dangerous positions such as against a hot radiator. Or fall asleep with their arm hanging over the back of a chair and sustain a paralysis of the axillary nerve. Many people assume that they go to sleep in a specific position and never move for eight hours – but actually you move much more than you think you do. Exactly how much is largely down to genes.* On average people move 13 times per hour with some people moving as many as 100 times an hour and others hardly at all.[40] You are highly unlikely to stay in the same position all night.

So, what about sleeping wrong? You go to bed fine and wake up with a stiff back or can't move your neck. It must be because you slept wrong. Right? Wrong! It's much more likely the reason for your back and neck pain is nothing to do with the conditions you slept under given you've done that hundreds of nights without a problem, but because your body was trying to repair something at night that has been brewing for a while. Inflammation is more active at night when we are injured and one of the clinical signs of inflammation is stiffness in the morning for longer than 30–40 minutes. It's more likely that something in your daily life has overloaded your back or neck and the consequences are now starting to show. If you are going through a stressful period or living a stressful life or not getting adequate sleep, you'll be more inflamed and therefore stiffer in the morning. It's not the pillow or mattress; it's your health hexagon being out of balance. As we have already seen, your body will let you know if things aren't working and one of its methods is to make you painful.

Liam bought seven mattresses over three years, trying to find the perfect one to ease his stiff back and neck. He had all the blood tests and imaging available to rule out inflammatory arthropathy. He came to see me every four to six months with flare-ups of back pain, despite being diligent about his flexibility

---

* A genetic marker called BTBD9 has been identified as affecting sleep movement.

and fitness routine. Typically, he came after one of his short trips to France. After purchasing numerous mattresses both at home and in France and getting similar results, he started blaming the seats of the low-cost airline he used. He had no such problems flying to South Africa, which he did every year and which was a much longer flight. It didn't make sense, but he was convinced.

I was sure he must have been under some sort of stress that was driving his HPA axis, stimulating a low-grade inflammation. Liam, however, like many high achievers I see, didn't believe he was feeling stressed because he wasn't feeling the emotional side effects that he thought indicated stress – feeling overwhelmed, anxious, nervous and afraid. That is true for many people but not all. For some people stress might look like high blood pressure, hives, irritable bowel or pain. Most often in my world it's pain.

After some time, Liam revealed that he was dealing with a very difficult family situation. Every time he went to France to deal with this situation, he was under enormous stress. Not just during their time in France but in the days leading up to it and around the days following their return. This was causing his HPA axis to produce cortisol, his inflammatory system to be primed, his sleep cycle to be disturbed. All of this was increasing his pain sensitivity. Some simple back stiffness turns into more aggressive back pain, but as we already know, persistent pain is not a reliable indicator of tissue harm or damage. Liam didn't link this family crisis in France with his pain. Seven mattresses later and he had to accept that the mattress wasn't responsible. His plane theory didn't make sense either. Once the pattern was consistent and reproducible, Liam was able to accept that his pain was secondary to a stress event. He began using his health hexagon to help him cope, no more mattress or pillow purchases necessary.

A comfortable bed is a wonderful thing, especially when you are exhausted. Physical effort such as a hard day's manual labour or a strenuous workout can make you tired, but will it help you sleep?

Exercise and diet

The belief that exercise helps you sleep is pervasive, but believe it or not, there isn't much evidence to support this.[41] The main reason for limited evidence is that most studies looking at such things are carried out on "normal' sleepers",[42] excluding those on medication that might affect their sleep or who have a variety of sleep disorders.

What about the benefits of exercise to those who do have some sleep difficulties? The most common sleep problems are insomnia and sleep-disordered breathing (SDB). A study by Reid and colleagues showed that four months of aerobic training in older adults with insomnia significantly improved sleep quality and reduced daytime sleepiness and symptoms of depression.[43] A metanalysis of five studies showed that exercise training reduced the severity of obstructive sleep apnoea by 32 per cent without any significant change to BMI.[44] Twelve weeks of moderate-intensity aerobic and resistance exercises resulted in a 25 per cent reduction in obstructive sleep apnoea symptoms and self-reported improvements in sleep quality, depressive symptoms, fatigue and quality of life.[45,46] These studies have quite small sample sizes, so more research is required to understand the various variables within exercise to see what is or isn't significant. Poor sleep and increased daytime sleepiness was associated with reduced physical function in adults,[47] suggesting a two-way association between sleep and exercise. If you are sleeping poorly and you are tired, that probably means you are less likely to be physically active.

The time of day that you exercise may also have an impact on your sleep. This won't be universal, but exercising too close to bedtime may make it harder to fall asleep. Exercising vigorously close to bedtime could mean that your core body temperature is higher than usual and therefore slower to fall, which may delay the onset of sleep. It may be a trade-off, where you weigh up the benefits you get from the exercise versus a slight reduction in sleep quantity that night.

One last element to consider is the routine of your exercise. As exercise can be a great de-stressor, continuing with your normal exercise routine at times of stress is a healthy approach. If you need a good night's sleep such as before an exam, an interview or an important sports performance, think carefully about how much exercise is enough to help you balance your health hexagon. I used to think that athletes needed to rest before major sporting contests to conserve their energy before the big event. In fact they usually train the day before, not necessarily intensely but enough to keep things ticking over and to help them get a better night's sleep. No training usually means they are restless and more anxious and that leads to poorer quality sleep.

Finally, diet. Going to bed too full or too hungry can make for a poor night's sleep, but is there any evidence that what you eat influences your sleep? Restricting your calorie intake to 800 calories a day for a month has been shown to decrease the amount of deep NREM sleep and makes it more difficult to fall asleep.[48] A diet high in carbohydrate and low in fat for two days decreases the amount of NREM sleep at night but increases REM sleep dreaming in comparison to a low-carbohydrate, high-fat diet for two days. Four days of a high-sugar, high-carbohydrate diet that is low in fibre resulted in less REM sleep and more night-time awakenings.[49] Poor sleep quantity however will increase hunger and appetite and affect impulse control leading to higher calorie intake and less satisfaction from food, contributing to weight gain. Plus if you are trying to diet and have poor sleep quantity, you'll lose lean body mass rather than fat.[50] It's also worth remembering that poor sleep affects your cortisol levels and plays a role in developing and exacerbating type 2 diabetes.

Sleep hygiene

There are plenty of websites and books out there that will offer you advice on how to get a good night's sleep so I won't cover that here – I particularly like *Why We Sleep* by Matthew Walker, who provides a solid understanding of the importance of sleep and a deeper understanding of the science behind it.

What I hope you take from this chapter is that sleep is essential. Sleep helps you repair and prepare. It improves your memory and helps you process trauma and important emotional events so you can learn from experience and deal with the future. It helps you repair tissues from injury and strengthen your immune system to fight disease. It helps your stress system and improves your mood. Exercise won't necessarily make you sleep better if you sleep pretty well already, but it may help if you are sleeping poorly. If you sleep poorly, you are less likely to exercise. Poor sleep is linked to heart disease, type 2 diabetes, exacerbation of mental health problems and pain. Sleep is fundamental to your health hexagon. Everything else gets worse without it.

And after a good night's sleep? Breakfast.

CHAPTER 10

Diet

YOU ARE WHAT you eat, or so they say, but does everyone respond
the same way to what they eat? Surprise, surprise, the answer
is no. How we react to food varies from person to person. A
Canadian study which looked at the impact of overfeeding groups
of identical twins by 1,000 calories a day for 84 days revealed
similar weight gains within identical twin pairings but significant
differences between twin pairings, suggesting that genes have a
significant impact on how we process food and store excess calories.[1] Some sets of twins gained 4.3 kg over the study, while others
gained as much as 13.3 kg. There were differences in how weight
was gained, as either lean muscle mass or fat, and differences in
fat distribution as abdominal or visceral between sets of twins. It's
not as simple as calories in versus calories out.

In 2017 the UK government spent £5.2 million on their
flagship Change4Life campaign, which promotes healthy eating
and exercise.[2] The advertising spend for non-essential foods such
as crisps, confectioneries and alcohol is an estimated £1 billion
per year. It's not exactly a fair game. An advertising psychologist
once told me that there were eight different ways to advertise to
people. Although you might see through several such methods
and consciously decide not to fall for them, you may not even
realise the others are working on you. Everyone is susceptible to

advertising, no matter how clever you are. Eating well is difficult and takes willpower, but like everything in your hexagon, if you have a purpose and a sense of direction, you can ask yourself whether your eating habits align with that purpose.

My patient Aidan had a back problem exacerbated by his weight, which meant he was at risk of needing surgery. If he could manage to lose weight, he could avoid the need for an operation. He hated going to the gym and lacked the motivation to exercise, lose weight and improve his back strength. The solution was cake. We agreed that if Aidan could lose weight and build up his strength by working with a personal trainer, then he could switch his motivation to exercise from helping his back pain to exercising for cake. When he did achieve his aims, he carried on going to the gym but now he would go to his personal training sessions with a picture of the slice of cake he was going to have after that session. He would ask his PT to work the exact number of calories for that day's slice of cake. If he was working for a slice of carrot cake that was 415 calories, his PT would let him know when he had reached his goal. If that was mid-set, he'd drop the dumbbell and walk out of there and straight to the café. It was unorthodox, but it worked for him.

This chapter is not a prescription on the best diet or right and wrong foods. It's about figuring out what is enough for you in this area. Your diet not only provides the fuel to give you energy, repair systems and sustain background functions, but it also affects your physical health and your mental health. "Enough" looks different for everyone. The number of calories you need will depend on the number of calories you burn. If you are running a marathon, you will clearly need more than someone sitting in an office, but you know that already.

In this chapter we will look at the importance of diet in a wider context of your health rather than the specifics about particular foods, food groups or energy expenditure. We will cover the importance of hydration, fasting, standing, medicine, inflammation and moderation, but first let's look at that most primitive sense of all. Gut feeling.

The gut-brain axis

Ivan Petrovich Pavlov stumbled across classical conditioning in his famous salivating dog experiments, for which he won a Nobel Prize in 1904. In his experiments, Pavlov rang a bell when he gave dogs their food. In time the dogs learned to associate the sound of the bell with the anticipation of food and would salivate to the sound of the bell. This demonstrated a connection between a stimulus, an emotional response and the digestive system linking the brain and the gut in what is now known as the gut-brain axis (GBA). The GBA is a channel of communication between the gut's own nervous system (the enteric nervous system) and the central nervous system of the brain and spinal cord, the autonomic nervous system, the endocrine system and the immune system. It links the emotional and cognitive regions of the brain with the functions of the intestines. Have you ever felt butterflies in your stomach or had loose bowels when you were stressed or anxious? Recent evidence suggests the gut's microbiome plays an important role here.[3]

There are trillions of microorganisms in the gut – in fact ten times more microorganisms than there are cells in the human body. Disruptions of the microbiome are associated with allergies, autoimmune disease, metabolic disorders such as obesity and mental health conditions such as anxiety and depression. You have multiple microbiome communities in and on your body that are individual and specific to you. These microbiomes react to internal and external environmental stimuli to help your body achieve a healthy balance.

The enteric nervous system, containing some 100 million neurons in the gut wall, connects to the brain via the vagus nerve. Changes in the gut wall send messages to the brain to signal hunger, fullness, nausea and pain. The feedback from the gut via the spinal and vagus nerves to the brainstem also engages the hypothalamus, which manages appetite among other things. Stimulation of the vagus nerve from the brain to the gut is thought to have an anti-inflammatory function.* Reduced parasympathetic ("rest-and-digest") activity of the vagus nerve is associated with abnormal growth and relocation of bacteria, showing the influence the vagus nerve has on manufacturing and distributing bacteria in the microbiome.

Sustained activation of the HPA axis and increased cortisol levels have been linked to an increased permeability of the gut wall or "leaky gut", facilitating a pro-inflammatory state.† It is also hypothesised that alterations to the diversity and composition of gut microbiota may be a risk factor in developing depressive behaviours[4] and anxiety.[5] Ninety-five per cent of serotonin, which is a neurotransmitter important in mood regulation and gut mobility, is manufactured by gut mucosal enterochromaffin cells.[6] The gut bacteria have also been shown to produce and

---

* Vagus nerve stimulation has helped treat the inflammatory pathways that contribute to rheumatoid arthritis; see Ines Doko, Simeon Grazio, Frane Grubišić, and Ralph Zitnik, "[Vagal Nerve Stimulation in the Treatment of Patients with Rheumatoid Arthritis – Results through Day 84 Obtained at the Croatian Center of an International Pilot Study]", *Reumatizam* 63, no. 2 (2016): 1–8.

† With increased levels of tumour necrosis factor α, interferon-γ and IL-6. IL-6 is known to activate the HPA axis, contributing to a chronic stress response.

consume a wide range of neurotransmitters, including dopamine, norepinephrine and gamma-aminobutyric acid (GABA), further indicating a link between gut health and emotional well-being.[7] As far back as 400 BC, Hippocrates was credited with saying, "Let food be thy medicine and medicine be thy food."[8]

What you eat and how your body will respond to it varies for everyone. Just as your genes influence how you store and process food, so does your gut microbiome. There is evidence to suggest that this starts from the beginning of your life, and it is noticeable that the microbes found in babies' guts differ depending on whether they were born by natural delivery or C-section.[9] There are wildly varying opinions about diets, but the consensus is that a diverse gut microbiome is a good thing. A healthy gut biome will improve your mental health, your stress response systems and your immune system, as well as helping to lower your risk of type 2 diabetes and heart disease and other inflammatory conditions such as inflammatory bowel disease, inflammatory arthritis and pain.[10]

People regularly ask me for my opinion on the best diet for them to follow. Most want to diet to lose weight or change something about how food makes them feel. Typically, this is a short-term plan of action to achieve a particular goal. My belief is that the word "diet" itself is unhelpful. By definition it suggests something temporary. My philosophy – which is far from unique – is that you want a sustainable relationship with food. Diets typically involve restricting your calorie intake, which can suppress your metabolism. That means that when you go back to a normal calorie intake, you will store more calories: your metabolism has been depressed and has learned to store from the period of "famine". This often leads to sudden weight loss followed by sudden weight gain and a series of yo-yo diets. The restriction in calories also reduces the diversity of your gut biome, which is likely to affect your well-being in the long run.

I appreciate that for some people there may be many reasons to lose weight quickly – some research suggests this is more important in the short term, such as restricting calories to 800 a day as part of attempts to reverse type 2 diabetes.[11] The priority in that instance may be to lose that weight fast and then work on your gut biome for the long term.

People often use diet as a way of trying to control something in their life if other areas feel out of control. This might not be the best thing for you. Your diet plays a significant role in regulating your health and your mood, and restricting yourself to a narrow range of food groups could risk making things worse, not better. It's not simple; what works for one person won't necessarily work for another.

Whatever diet you might be considering, there's one thing that almost everyone agrees on. Diets high in sugar and processed foods are bad for our microbes. The evidence suggests that in general terms, gut biome diversity is reducing decade on decade. As we eat more and more high-sugar, low-fat, processed foods we also see a rise in autoimmune disease, allergies, diabetes and inflammatory conditions. So what to do? Well, diversity is key. Food and health writer Michael Pollan's sound advice is "don't eat anything your great-grandmother's microbes wouldn't recognise as food".[12] Ideally you want to get as many varieties of natural products into your diet as possible. Plenty of different vegetables, live cheeses and yogurts, seeds and nuts, olive oil and some fruit. Why not try tracking what you eat over an average week, fortnight or month, and looking at the variety of ingredients you are getting? You might be surprised at how few that really is.

Hydration

As we saw in the introduction to this book your body uses pain to guide or warn you, to help you pay attention and ultimately to protect you from harm. Sometimes it's hard to pay attention to those signs and systems, and dehydration is a good example of this.

Our bodies are 60 per cent water, and our brains are 90 per cent water. It's important to stay hydrated, so your body tries to help you achieve this. The first sign of dehydration might be that your urine is yellow. No pain at this point, just a physical sign that your hydration status isn't optimum. You might notice but you don't give it much attention. You feel OK. A short while later you realise you're thirsty. Your system is turning the signals up a notch to alert you that your hydration levels are reducing, but you're still too busy to act. Meetings, emails, places to go, people to see. No fluids consumed. Later still, your body needs to make you notice so it decides to give you a headache. Now you're becoming aware, but do you do the right thing? Of course not. You've got a headache; you must need a coffee or a painkiller with a sip of water.

You're busy and the headaches keep coming. You're stressed, there's too much going on. That's why you're getting a headache, right? Wrong. You haven't been paying attention. Your body tried to give you some obvious signs, but you didn't take in adequate fluids. An espresso is not the solution.

This pattern continues over several days. Now you're getting increasingly dehydrated and pain has to elevate its efforts further. There are only a few more places your pain system can go to warn you and here comes one of them: cramp.

Pain most definitely has your attention now. You'll jump around the place and stop what you're doing. But even then, will you do what it takes? Will you put a system in place to deal with this to prevent it happening again? You might drink some water, probably not enough, but at least you're thinking about it. Tomorrow is another day and you put that cramp down to "just one of those things".

Carry on like this over weeks and months and your pain system is going to have to go nuclear. There are consequences to ignoring the signs. Your body was trying to protect you from what's coming next. A kidney stone and a whole world of pain.

Ask anyone who has had kidney stones. They make sure they drink plenty of fluids after that. Now if they see that their urine is yellow, they are terrified, for a while at least, that they might be getting another kidney stone.

Having yellow urine doesn't mean you need to go into hospital and be put on a drip, but it does mean you need to take a drink. It does mean you need to put a system in place to make sure you do drink adequately every day, and you do need to take responsibility for it. It's important to make sure you are measuring the correct metric. It's OK to have yellow urine from time to time provided you "wee white once a day". (Well, pale yellow really, but "wee white" is easier to remember.) Don't panic when you do have yellow urine. Instead, see it as motivation.

Hopefully you don't need to go as far as getting kidney stones to motivate you to drink, but if you do need a reason or two to make sure you have at least a glass of water with every meal, here are a few good ones. Water helps you flush out waste products via your kidneys; it helps you digest your food, improves your skin, lubricates your joints and muscles, cushions your brain and spinal cord. It helps regulate hormones and temperature and boosts your mental capacity.

When you start to feel thirsty, most likely you are already dehydrated by 1–2 per cent. That might not sound like a lot, but 1–2 per cent can affect your concentration levels and your short-term and working memory, as well as delay reaction times and cause moodiness and anxiety.[13] Even after rehydrating, the effects on fatigue, vigour and mood persist.[14] Physical performance has also been shown to decline with dehydration as measured in sports such as basketball, resulting in progressively reduced accuracy, slower shooting time and increased number of shots. In surfing dehydration has been linked to a 20.3 per cent reduction in performance, and in golf it's been shown to contribute to a reduction in ball carry, shot accuracy and distance judgement.[15]

Most of us don't consider water to be a nutrient, but it is a vital one. Dehydration causes an increased heart rate due to the lower viscosity of the blood, putting the body into a state of stress. Dehydration can also cause difficulty with thermoregulation. Sweating is part of your body's ability to release heat: if you don't have the fluid to lose, you will increase core body temperature. This could also affect your ability to fall asleep. Your fluid intake contributes to your calorie consumption, with some studies showing a reduction in total energy intake of 10–13 per cent by switching from carbonated flavoured drinks, juice and whole milk to water.[16] Studies have also shown that those who drink water before a meal consume fewer calories.[17] As hunter-gatherers, without reliable access to clean drinking water, we would have obtained a lot of our hydration from food. Now you might feel hungry when in fact you're thirsty. Consider this the next time you go to grab a snack. Maybe it's water you need, not carbs.

You will get your fluids from many sources – food, water, hot drinks, juice, milk. How you take your fluids will affect your hydration. Some studies suggest milk allows you to retain more of the fluid you consume: it has calories that water hasn't, but it also has calcium, unlike water.[18] Choices, choices! Tea and coffee are fine in moderation, but you will reach a point where you're taking in too much caffeine. After consuming about 500 milligrams of caffeine in a day it becomes a diuretic, where you lose more water than it gives you.[19]

More isn't necessarily better when it comes to fluids, though. Too much fluid can leave you suffering from hyponatraemia where the levels of sodium in your blood are diluted, with significant health consequences. Occasionally it can even be fatal. Scenarios where you take on large amounts of water, such as endurance events, can also be a risk. A study of the 2002 Boston Marathon showed that 13 per cent of participants experienced hyponatraemia.[20] Clinical signs of hyponatraemia include nausea, vomiting, headache, confusion, loss of energy, drowsiness, fatigue, irritability, muscle cramps, spasms and in severe cases seizures and coma. Too little or too much are both problematic. The key is enough.

The amount of fluid you need will vary from day to day. Although the European Food Safety Authority recommends 2.5 L per day for men and 2 L per day for women, it depends on what you do and where you are.[21,22] You lose water through sweat, breathing and urination. The climate, how much you exercise and how much you are breathing will all affect your fluid balance. If you're used to having a jug of water on your desk during the working week you may be taking in enough water, but do you end up drinking less over the weekend because it's not there? Weeing white once a day is a simple guideline but so is the number of times you go to the toilet per day. Fewer than four times is too little, more than eight is probably too many.[23]

Given that we all know that without water we will die within days, why isn't it higher on our priority lists? It's really not that hard to fill a jug a day and work your way through it or have a glass with every meal. Your energy levels will be better, your concentration and decision-making will improve, you'll be more alert, your skin will look healthier, you'll have fewer headaches and your kidneys will thank you for it too.

Thinking fast and slow

Your body has evolved to follow circadian rhythms such as your sleep-wake cycle. Your digestive system follows a similar diurnal rhythm to prepare your body for predictable availability of nutrients during the normal feeding period. Among other things, this helps to optimise your gastrointestinal digestion and regulate glucose, lipids and bile acid metabolism.[24] Eating late into the night or close to bed unsettles this system. Melatonin, which is released as a trigger for sleep, decreases insulin secretion. That means that the food you eat late at night won't be digested properly and could lead to higher blood glucose levels, contributing to the risk of diabetes.[25] Eating late and delaying sleep are associated with obesity, metabolic dysregulation and raised inflammatory markers.[26] Snacking before bed typically involves unnecessary calories high in fat and sugar.

Time-restricted eating (TRE) involves a period of 12–14 hours without food in a 24-hour day. For example, you might not eat anything from 7 p.m. until 9 a.m. the next day. The research suggests that this can significantly improve blood glucose regulation, reducing your risk of diabetes and fatty liver disease and lowering blood pressure and cholesterol. It may even contribute to weight loss, without changing the number of calories you eat.[27] TRE also allows the gut to cleanse itself and reduces mucous in the bowel as well as contributing to a more restful sleep.[28,29] In fasting mode the body moves from burning glucose to ketones, which the liver produces from fat. During a period of fasting, the body goes into survival and repair mode and then switches into growth and regeneration after feeding when back in the glucose phase of energy production or usage. It's believed that this can help with brain cell regeneration, provide resilience to neurological conditions, and slow the effects of aging.[30]

Plant-based foods and drinks rich in polyphenols[31] have been shown to affect cognitive health as well as fruit and vegetables,[32] nuts, whole grains and legumes[33,34,35] and coffee.[36] Sitting buried in the office surrounded by paperwork and grabbing a highly processed, high-sugar lunch might be quick and easy, but is it worth the price of admission?

Stand up to glucose

A group of 800 people had their blood glucose monitored every five minutes over a week. Half of them were overweight, a quarter obese and the remainder a healthy weight – to replicate the non-diabetic population of the Western world. This study covered 46,898 meals with ten million calories logged.[37] The researchers discovered huge variability in how individuals responded to foods. For some, their blood glucose was significantly elevated by eating ice cream while for others it had no effect. Some had high blood glucose after eating sushi while others reacted to nectarines, milk or tomatoes. The individual variabilities were dramatic, showing that not everyone is the same and a "diet" suitable for one is not suitable for everyone.

This research group also looked at individual gut biomes: they found they could predict how people would react to certain foods with surprising accuracy by analysing their gut biome first and matching it to specific foods in a study of an additional 100 people.[38] Most of us won't have a glucose monitor or gut biome test on hand to figure out how we react to every food, but I can see a day where it becomes routine.

What do you do after you eat? Research suggests standing after you eat helps you digest food better and can help reduce blood glucose, thus reducing your risk of type 2 diabetes.[39,40] It may also reduce cholesterol.[41] A sit-stand desk may well be a better idea than sitting down all day. Not only will it help your blood sugars, but it also contributes to weight-bearing, which stimulates your bones to be stronger. Better still, get out and have a walk. You might get some sunshine, which gives you vitamin D. This essential vitamin helps build your bones, improves inflammatory markers[42] and boosts your immune system.[43] We all feel better for a walk in the sunshine and vitamin D deficiency is considered a factor in depression.[44] You can get vitamin D from some foods, such as swordfish, tuna, salmon, cod liver oil, egg yolks and sardines, but you'll get the majority from sunshine no matter how much you eat so get outside every day. It will help your sleep, digestion, inflammatory markers, immune system and stress levels. Just being outside counts but of course I'll say move while you're at it.

What about supplements? you might ask. That's next.

Medication and supplements

The diet element of your hexagon includes appropriate medications. After all, this is something you put into your body just like food. When it comes to supplements, I'm not going to tell you which supplements are beneficial and which ones are a waste of time: I'll leave you to do your own research on that and what's right for you. What I will say though is don't dismiss them. I see a lot of patients who are reluctant to try any medicines, believing that they are all somehow bad or unnecessary. I'm not qualified to prescribe and I don't purport to know what works for what, but I do know that they absolutely have their place.

Yes, people can be overprescribed drugs for everything and anything. Yes, some medications are necessary at certain stages of a condition and no longer work at other stages of a condition. Yes, some people struggle with dependency and some people have more side effects than others. Yes, some medications work better for some people and others are allergic. Enough is different for each of us. Sometimes enough of something for you will be zero and sometimes enough might be a week of antibiotics for that chest infection, which could turn into pneumonia if you don't get on top of it. Sometimes enough is a number of medications every day for the rest of your life. My point is, don't dismiss anything out of hand.

Often resistance appears in the context of antidepressants or medication for other mental health conditions. As is now abundantly clear, each aspect of your hexagon is linked to your overall physical and mental well-being, and imbalance in one area can affect another in complex ways. Serotonin plays a significant role in your pain system and it's therefore no surprise that people with a history of depression experience more pain while people in persistent pain are more likely to become depressed.[45] A family of antidepressant medications called selective serotonin reuptake inhibitors (SSRIs) work on regulating serotonin and can be helpful in certain circumstances for certain people – if you think that might include you, talk to your doctor.

Approximately 95 per cent of serotonin is made in the gut so a healthy digestive system matters.

Because carbohydrates are involved in synthesising a derivative of serotonin called 5-HT,[46] craving foods high in carbohydrates and fats, like crisps or pastries, could indicate that your serotonin levels aren't optimum.[47] That is not to say that if you fancy a sandwich or a packet of crisps, you must be depressed; but if you are comfort eating, gaining weight, craving carbs, feeling remorseful or pessimistic and not sleeping well, maybe you need some professional help to get your serotonin levels right before you can focus on any part of your hexagon.

Obesity and depression often go together. Of course, depression isn't exclusive to obesity and being obese doesn't mean you will be or are depressed. In Chapter 8 on the spiritual space, we looked at how injury and stress can lead to inflammation, which can lead to depression. Excess adipose tissue (fat) has a high density of cells such as macrophages (responsible for a pro-inflammatory response) and interleukin 6, which is known to stimulate your stress system, the HPA axis.[48]

Inflammation is a killer. You sleep poorly, you get inflamed. You push yourself too hard, you get inflamed. You do too little, you get inflamed. You get injured, you get inflamed. You get stressed, you get inflamed. Stress makes us more likely to eat unhealthy foods and make unhealthy choices. Unhealthy choices can make you obese, and obesity makes your inflammatory system more active. The cycle becomes ever harder to break. This is the whole purpose of the health hexagon in a nutshell: to recognise the connections between your biology, your stress system, a pro-inflammatory lifestyle and the choices you make that construct your hexagon.

Moderation

It's not all bad. You don't have to live like a monk from the fifteenth century. Enough is what matters. My father used to say, "Everything in moderation, including moderation itself." Shocking your digestive system from time to time can actually help to keep it on its toes.[49] If your gut biome isn't challenged every now and again it can get lazy, so the occasional fried breakfast or BBQ blowout could be helpful. If nothing else, they might remind you why you tend to avoid certain foods in the first place as they make you feel rubbish, and that helps reacquaint you with your purpose.

If you're looking for something with a scientific stamp of approval, the evidence suggests there are health benefits from a chemical compound called flavonoids, found in strawberries, tea, onions, blueberries, apples and cocoa. The concentration of flavonoids is high in dark chocolate, and the darker the better. Researchers have found that eating a couple of squares of dark chocolate daily can improve the elasticity of blood vessels, reduce blood pressure, improve insulin sensitivity and improve cholesterol levels. It can even improve the blood supply to your brain, thereby helping cognition. Researchers believe that flavonoids are converted by your gut bacteria into smaller anti-inflammatory compounds that can pass through the blood-brain barrier and may have a neuroprotective effect.[50]

Coffee also has some proven health benefits. A review of 201 studies on the subject published in the *British Medical Journal* in 2017 found that drinking coffee lowered the risk of heart disease and cancer most likely because of its antioxidant and anti-inflammatory properties.[51] Coffee also had favourable results when it came to Alzheimer's disease and Parkinson's disease.

But how much is enough? We know that after 500 mg, caffeine starts to become a diuretic, so beyond that it offers diminishing returns from a hydration perspective. A cup of instant coffee contains between 60 and 80 mg of caffeine and brewed filter coffee between 60 and 120 mg. Two to five cups a day is considered enough in terms of hydration and the reported health benefits I've mentioned. It may also be worth noting that your ability to process coffee depends on a particular genetic marker, CYP1A2, which controls a liver enzyme that helps break down caffeine. If you have it, you'll metabolise caffeine quicker than those who don't possess that gene.

There is no one-size-fits-all diet so be wary of the latest craze. Your gut biome is yours and yours alone. Its health has a significant impact on your weight, your energy levels, your immune system, your inflammatory system and both your physical and psychological well-being. Diversity is key and processed food is not good. Stay hydrated: your brain is relying on you to keep it that way and it has many ways of helping you stay on track. Having a clear sense of purpose will help you stay disciplined in choosing what and when to eat. The occasional blowout is OK. As always, be careful who you compare yourself to.

CHAPTER 11

Stored Data

YOUR BRAIN IS your command centre, and it remembers everything. Every experience you've had, everything you've heard, everything you've seen, everything you've inherited. Some of it you can access easily and some of it is buried in places that are harder to get to. A lot of the work it does is automatic: you don't even realise it's happening.

Each time you gather some information, your brain will file it away into various departments that have developed through millions of years of evolution to deal with every aspect of your being. When you encounter a stimulus, your brain searches through these departments to find the information relevant to it to help you decide how to react.

Much of this decision-making happens through an area of the brain known as the limbic system, which deals with the more emotional aspects of your being. The prefrontal cortex is the executive centre of the brain that deals with planning, decision-making and the ability to regulate your behaviour in line with social norms. Think of it like a boardroom of a major corporation. Each department of the limbic system gives its opinion on a situation, and the chairperson is the prefrontal cortex, which can elicit top-down control over the other board members. These regions or members of the board negotiate with each other to decide what is in your best interests at any moment. Of course, they can only do so with the information they have available. When you're under stress, it's more difficult for your prefrontal cortex to negotiate with your limbic system;[1] your reactions can end up being more instinctive than logical and not necessarily appropriate for the situation you are in, or in your best interests in the long run.

The stimuli you experience can be positive and negative. Your reactions to those stimuli can also be positive or negative, and will be influenced by many biological and environmental factors. You may react differently to the same stimulus if you are hungry or tired than you would if you were not. Your decision-making process could be very different after a bottle of wine than after a cup of tea. The information you already hold internally as stored data will influence how you behave; how you use those stored data will depend on which parts of your brain win the negotiation. Your brain is plastic and capable of learning: if you are aware of how you react to different situations, you can use the different departments of your brain and the information you hold to change your behaviour and choose different outcomes for yourself.

In this chapter we'll take a quick look at some of the brain's departments and what they are responsible for. They are all interconnected and so don't operate in isolation, but we will try to separate and organise the different areas for simplicity and to show what the relevance of each brain area might be for your pain experience.

Reception area

The **thalamus** is the relay centre where sensory information arriving in the brain is sent on to various regions of the cerebral cortex to be considered. Think of it like the reception area of your brain

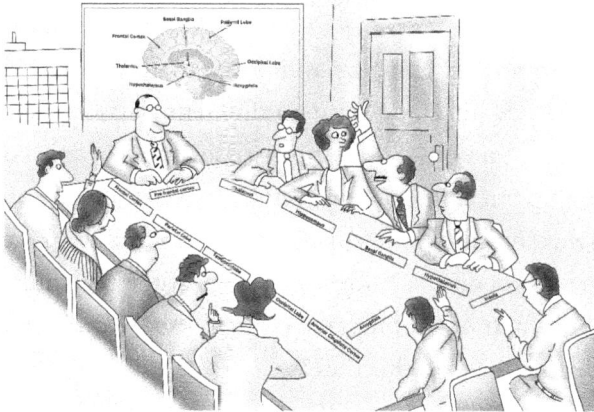

Figure 3: Stored Data
The brain represented as a boardroom with each department of
the brain giving their opinion on the situation. A negotiation
takes place between the board members (limbic system) and
the chairperson (pre-frontal cortex) to make a decision.

or a switchboard that receives incoming sensory messages and then directs them to the appropriate brain departments. It acts as the first filter or check-point, providing some preliminary processing of signals before they reach the cortex.

The thalamus has various relay nuclei,[2] which receive messages from specific sources to help it pass information on to the appropriate department. In basic terms these relay nuclei take messages from specific inputs and direct them to specific brain areas. Different nuclei connect to different parts of the brain. Some of them pass on sensory input, such as touch, smell or proprioception (your ability to sense action, movement and position); others relay auditory and visual signals, emotional processing, memory and cognition. A message arrives at the thalamus and is directed to a part of the brain which says: "Ah, yeah. I remember this. What shall we do this time?"

Habit

The few milliseconds between thought and action are crucial to decision-making. The **basal ganglia** are a group of nuclei that form part of the planning mechanism for movement; they work with the frontal lobe and cingulate cortex to select appropriate motor responses.[3] The basal ganglia are responsible for habit learning. Damage to the basal ganglia can result in uncontrollable movements. Part of the basal ganglia, the claustrum, is thought to filter out "unnecessary" sensory stimuli to focus on what is important or salient. The thalamus, by contrast, directs attention to a broad range of stimuli. Salience is based on past experience and depends on your personal motivation or purpose.

The basal ganglia rely on old rules when presented with familiar environmental and context stimuli. It is up to the cortex to alter a learned response or habit. In persistent pain you can very quickly attach significance to objects or situations that you believe are important to your pain experience. Perhaps after a foot or ankle injury you found certain shoes more comfortable than others. As you healed this information became less relevant, but you held on to the belief that shoes have a significant impact on your pain. The information may no longer be appropriate by this stage in your recovery, but you haven't updated your cortex accordingly to help the basal ganglia and other regions alter your learned response. You fixate on shoes being "good" or "bad" and avoid doing things that are good for you because you believe you can't wear the appropriate shoes for the job. You don't hike because you can't wear walking boots, or you don't dress up for a wedding because you can no longer wear heels – you still go but you feel awkward and isolated because you don't feel you're dressed properly. Your brain is filtering messages on old data: somewhere along the line you were told not to wear high heels and no one you trusted ever said it was OK to start wearing heels again.

Memory retrieval

New memories are stored in part of the **hippocampus** called the CA3 field. Later they are consolidated into long-term memory in neocortical or new memory storage areas in the brain. The hippocampus keeps a small part of the memory or memory tag within the CA3 field to help it retrieve the entire memory from the neocortex when required. The CA1 field of the hippocampus looks for similarities in your current situation with memory tags stored in the CA3 field. When it recognises similarities, it can trigger the retrieval of the entire previous experience to complete a pattern in the CA3 field.[4] You can end up using snippets of data to fill in the gaps to predict what you should see or do.

Many optical illusions work this way. You anticipate seeing a triangle as the image looks very similar, so your brain fills in the gaps; but when you look closely the triangle may not be complete. You will do this with pain too. The CA1 field is linked to autobiographical memory.[5] You might have a snippet of memory that something was painful in a past experience. When faced with a similar situation again, this shapes your prediction of what will happen. Your body then reacts to defend itself.

This is not to say that the hippocampus is entirely responsible for your reaction. What's important to understand is that various regions of the brain use data to see what's significant from their point of view; this will be used alongside the other areas to eventually come up with a reaction. Different departments of the brain carry different influence or weighting over a decision depending on how powerful the association is. The negotiation that takes place among these departments will determine your response and your future behaviour.

Have you ever surprised yourself by recalling the lyrics of a song you haven't heard for years? A snippet of the opening bars can be enough to pull out the entire song from your memory bank. This can happen with a persistent pain experience too. Think of pain like a piece of music that you are exposed to. You don't necessarily like the song but it's everywhere. It's constantly on the radio, on TV, in ads and movies. It's a huge hit, a cultural phenomenon. Your brain will store that song and have a memory for it. You will associate it with a certain period in your life, perhaps a particular job or house, a partner, a friend.

Eventually the song fades away and you won't be consciously aware of it, but it doesn't take much to trigger your memory. Perhaps years later someone whistles it as they walk past or someone makes a reference to a movie the song was in and it comes flooding back instantly. Not just the song, but anything you associate with it. Places, people, situations, emotions. Persistent pain acts in a similar way. If that pain has been following you around for more than three months, it will have built a very strong memory in your brain, and it might not take much to trigger the pain down the line. We'll explore this a bit more when we come to neurotags in Chapter 12.

Risk/reward

The **amygdala** monitors internal and external sensory triggers, but its main function is a danger detector. The amygdala matches sensory input with emotions and decides on the reward value of a specific stimulus.[6] If you are walking in the jungle, a rattle sound could indicate a venomous snake. If you are in a toy shop, it's more likely to be a toy rattle and less likely to be dangerous. The same stimulus but very different interpretations based on environment, experience and likely outcome. When you see a new face, you will use both the hippocampus and the amygdala to decide whether it is likely to be friend or foe. Although the amygdala is associated with fear and anxiety, it is also activated by positive stimulus. The hippocampus and the amygdala are critical in forming memories and associating surroundings or context with pleasurable situations.

The anterior hippocampus is the centre of personal emotional memory. It can influence the emotional experience elicited by the amygdala to a stimulus as both structures are simultaneously activated when you remember emotional events.[7] In persistent pain terms this can mean old memories come flooding back as a result of sensory cues that you have not been exposed to for years. For example, a smell reminds you of a traumatic time where you got injured, which then leads to the various parts of the brain making that old, injured body part more vigilant and waking up some pain pathways. A smell could equally remind you of a positive time and flood you with warm nostalgia.

Visual input is particularly powerful in humans. Signals from the visual cortex can reach the amygdala before the cerebral cortex is aware of what's happening.[8] Subliminal stimuli that arrive this way can account for the phenomenon of blindsight or sixth sense. This can cause the amygdala to initiate a defence response milliseconds before the cortex is aware it's happening. The amygdala connects directly to the HPA axis[9] so if the amygdala associates a stimulus with danger, this could mean you go into a stress response before you have had a chance to consider the situation intellectually. Your HPA axis has already reacted instinctively before you've had a chance to rationalise what's going on. On occasion you can use the higher centres of the brain to negotiate and moderate your response.

In persistent pain terms it is possible to have a reflexive response to a stimulus you are not even aware you are reacting to. By the time you have gone into defensive mode with a guarded muscular response (which itself can produce pain), it's easy to associate the pain with whatever you are doing at that moment. You then start to associate that activity with danger even though it may not be dangerous.

Let's say you hurt your back in a game of rugby. While you were injured, lots of things were painful. As you improved some things were painful, and some things were fine. One day you were feeling pretty good and you bent down to put something into the dishwasher. Your back suddenly went into spasm, putting you out of action for a couple of days. It was frustrating and it rattled your confidence: you thought you were doing much better than that. Now you start to see stacking the dishwasher as a dangerous activity. Why you got pain at that precise moment is probably more complicated than that. Perhaps you were tired or stressed; perhaps you were somehow inflamed and your nociceptors were hypervigilant; perhaps the kids were being annoying, and you were running late for work.

Any number of things could have primed your pain pathway, but because you got pain while loading the dishwasher, the dishwasher now starts to represent a threat. Even though by this point you have returned to the gym and got back to playing rugby, your amygdala continues to see the dishwasher as dangerous. This doesn't make sense. Putting a plate into a dishwasher is not a challenge to your spine when you're capable of playing rugby with a lot of physical contact, bending and twisting. Unfortunately your amygdala and hippocampus don't see it that way unless they are updated. It's a form of classical conditioning like Pavlov's dog.

You will have thousands of associations that influence your behaviour subliminally without you ever being aware of them. A 2012 study in the *Journal of Personality and Social Psychology* looked at the effect of the smell of fish in a room on players who were participating in a game with a partner. The game involved the player investing money with a partner in anticipation of their success and likely return on the player's investment. In the presence of the smell of fish, players in a game reduced their investment by 25 per cent. They became less likely to send money to their partner because they didn't trust their partner to share their profits later in the game. Other bad odours didn't have the same effect; only the smell of fish.

We use the phrase "something smells fishy" to indicate suspicion. The smell of fish makes you suspicious and subliminally influences your behaviour. It's also been shown that if you are suspicious about something, you are more sensitive to the smell of fish. This was probably helpful from an evolutionary point of view that you were able to identify safe or dangerous food by its smell. In time this turned into associating "fishy" with suspicion. Cultural associations will influence the negotiation that takes place within your brain and therefore also your behaviour.[10,11]

The amygdala responds quickly to environmental cues, leading to short-term responses such as the startle response, which is usually accompanied by the immediate sense of short-term fear. The higher cognitive centres of the brain, such as the orbitofrontal and ventromedial prefrontal cortices, establish reward/punishment values and propose activities that operate longer than the short-term responses controlled by the amygdala. The amygdala reacts while the cerebral cortex continually updates the context, including objects, rules, actions and sense of self, providing a source of control over the amygdala. Think of the jockey who falls off a horse and breaks their ankle but in the circumstances is relieved that they haven't been paralysed. The context will contribute to the reaction.

Failure of the prefrontal top-down control of the amygdala has been proposed as a contributor to anxiety disorders, major depression, PTSD and panic disorders.[12] Highly anxious people have weaker fibre connections between the amygdala and prefrontal and ventromedial cortices.[13] If you tend to be very anxious, then organising your health hexagon may help you see that your pain flares up in scenarios that challenge your personality. Think of the introverted scientist trying to be an extroverted social net-worker. Such situations make it harder for your prefrontal cortex to negotiate with your amygdala, heightening the activity of the HPA axis and priming your pain system.

With persistent pain, because there are so many subliminal classical conditioning connections being made in those first three months of an injury and beyond, you have to question whether your pain actually makes sense. Does it really make sense that putting a cup into a dishwasher could be bad for your back when you are doing Russian twists in the gym with a 25 kg kettlebell? The pain experience is real, but is it appropriate and necessary? Your pain pathway may be generating a response that isn't appropriate for the action you are doing, so something else must be going on. Perhaps it's activated because of other factors, such as stress or a learned response or a pro-inflammatory lifestyle. Pain is trying to tell you something, just not necessarily what you might assume it is.

Conscious awareness

The **anterior cingulate cortex** (ACC) connects to the amygdala, hypothalamus, brainstem and ventral striatum. It is the emotional division of the cingulate cortex, providing the motivation to carry out selected behaviours.[14] This is where the brain enters a conscious state of target selection. The ACC helps predict the consequences of an action through its connections with the lateral prefrontal cortex and plays an important role in self-regulation.[15]

The ACC evaluates incoming emotion-provoking stimuli and helps decide the most appropriate response. It receives input

181

from the amygdala, which prompts it to make a decision, a call to action. The prefrontal cortex negotiates with both areas and can exert control over the ACC and the amygdala, which has a bias towards danger or negativity to influence an outcome.[16] This doesn't suppress the amygdala's activity, however, which means you may be left with an ongoing enhanced feeling of fear and anxiety.

Think of this like performance anxiety before a speech. You feel anxious, nervous and fearful but you tell yourself you can do this, you know your subject, the audience are not hostile and you are the expert in the room. You suppress the urge to run away, and you go ahead and start. You have used top-down control from the executive centre of your brain, the prefrontal cortex, to suppress the influence of the amygdala and anterior cingulate cortex that were making you feel anxious and like you wanted to quit. Although your heart may race and your voice wobble slightly as you begin, chances are you'll settle into it pretty quickly. You might even find you enjoy it.

You need to do something similar when it comes to persistent pain. When you have persistent pain, you stop doing things that are good for you because you fear the pain you are experiencing means they are harming you. Let's say you hurt your back lifting some heavy weights in the gym. You now know that beyond three months, the pain is no longer a reliable indicator that you have damaged tissue. If you haven't understood the healing process, didn't have help with rehabilitating and had a lot of negative information reinforced within you while you were in the early stages of injury/recovery, your pain system's parking sensors get better and better at protecting you. Before long you are finding that you are doing less and less in order to avoid pain. You get to the stage where you no longer bring the bins out because that's a form of lifting. This makes you increasingly fearful and it also makes you stiffer, weaker and more likely to stimulate pain. Avoiding action is making things worse, not better.

What you see

The occipital lobe at the back of the brain is exclusively involved in processing what you see.[17] This gives you a huge amount of context to orientate yourself. Your eyes move all the time, jumping from one thing to another to help you figure out the most important thing to focus on at any point. Visual targets compete for your attention and the emotional aspects of what you see direct your attention while simultaneously suppressing other distractions.

For example, when you are trying to pick out a face in a crowd your brain will imagine the face you are looking for and scan the room for that face while trying to blank out others. This is why a scene might seem like a blur and then the face you are looking for pops into focus. What you see gives you a frame of reference not only for where you are and what you focus on but also for what you overlook or dismiss – and this will influence what you feel, how you think, what you anticipate and what you remember. What you miss can be just as important, if not more so, as what you see.

The famous Harvard gorilla experiment is a good example of this phenomenon.[18] In 1999 Christopher Chabris and Daniel Simons conducted an experiment to demonstrate selective attention. They showed some Harvard students a video of two teams of basketball players, one team dressed in white and the other in black. These students, among the brightest in the country, were naturally keen to impress their professors. They were asked to count the number of times the team in white successfully passed the ball to each other during the 25-second video clip. At the end of the video, they were asked for the number of successfully completed passes. The correct answer was 15. The professors then asked, "What about the gorilla?" Approximately halfway through the video a person dressed in a gorilla suit walks into shot, bangs their chest a few times and walks on. Half of the students didn't even notice. Their attention was fixed on the white team passing the ball: as far as they were concerned, everything else was out of focus or wasn't necessary to consider. When shown the video again, these students couldn't believe they had missed the gorilla. They were convinced it was a different video.

In pain terms your brain will remember visual clues that it associates with pain and give them emotional significance. If your back hurts when sitting down, your brain will attach emotional relevance to chairs and you will be vigilant as to which chairs are more comfortable than others. When you walk into a room with different seating options, you will seek out the chair that your brain imagines to be the best for your back. You will apportion emotional bias to certain chairs and if you don't get the one you want, you are likely to feel uncomfortable more quickly. You will pay more attention to how your back feels and are likely to feel frustrated that you didn't get the chair you wanted. This is likely to reinforce your belief that there are good chairs and bad chairs, further strengthening the pathways that process that information and making them more likely to repeat this process in the future. You are so focused on finding the right chair and on feeling irritable when you don't that you miss the gorilla in the room. In this context, the gorilla is gravity. Gravity will have the same effect on every chair in the room and therefore the chairs are all more or less the same. It doesn't really matter which chair you sit on.

Of course some chairs are more comfortable than others, but one chair is no more dangerous than another; that's an important difference to register. In persistent pain it's very common to fixate on a particular piece of information – such as that there are chairs that are good for your back and ones that will do you damage. If that information is not questioned and challenged using all available evidence, it becomes a belief system that shapes your pain experience.

Nancy was a surgeon who came to see me about persistent back pain. She had this exact same issue with "good" and "bad" chairs. It took some time but eventually we found a way to help her understand that a fixation on good and bad chairs wasn't reliable. We identified a scenario where the same type of chair was found in two different work-related situations: their outpatient clinic and management meetings. Nancy eventually worked out that her back became painful sooner in a management meeting than during an outpatient clinic. Her tolerance for sitting was lower in a management meeting. If the chair alone was responsible for her back pain, that same chair ought to produce the same result in any situation – but it didn't. I asked her why she thought her back hurt more in a management meeting. The penny dropped. She hated management meetings.

Once Nancy registered that there was more to her pain than the binary fixed mindset of good and bad chairs, she started to look at things differently. She stopped putting more emphasis on a chair than was necessary and accepted that chairs in themselves weren't dangerous. She started training her pain system to deal with different types of chairs and negotiated with her pain system by identifying enjoyable situations where she could sit for hours without a problem, such as long drives, the cinema, a pub with friends, a nice meal. During management meetings and outpatient clinics, she was able to negotiate with herself to dial down her vigilance about the chair. She focused on her health hexagon as a solution rather than blaming the chair.

In persistent pain it is very common to attach emotional significance to pieces of information that will influence how you behave and therefore how you feel. We will explore this more in Chapter 12. The problem is that your stored data can only filter through the information it has. You need to pay attention to all available information so that where relevant, you can update your stored data with the relevant new information. This can change your filtering process, which in turn changes your pain experience. You no longer look at something and anticipate it will be painful because you have updated your stored data.

If you do look at something and anticipate it is going to hurt, you will brace yourself. That's where the parietal lobe comes in.

Making a move

The **parietal lobe** responds continually to your environment and to sensory signals such as touch, temperature and proprioception. It is involved with body image and spatial awareness by predicting the weight, speed, location and distance of the objects around you.[19] It helps you tell the difference between left and right. It is part of the brain's attention centres,[20] which are responsible for directing your attention towards external stimuli ("Is that my phone ringing?") or important and unexpected prompts ("Did I unplug the iron?").

Signals from the parietal lobe communicate with signals from the visual, auditory and vestibular systems to allow you to plan your interactions in the world. The **precuneus** is a part of the parietal lobe that constantly monitors your peripheral visual fields and can draw your attention to a new target at any point in time. It is also involved in reflective thinking, mind-wandering or day-dreaming. This area of the brain is active when you are preparing to move or when you are moving in space, such as reaching or pointing. It activates when you are thinking about movement even if no movement is being made.[21] The frontal lobe can inhibit the precuneus, making it less active so you can focus on a task and avoid distractions. Think of the basketball/gorilla experiment. By focusing on the task of counting successful passes, the frontal lobe dialled down the precuneus's activity, making it more difficult to monitor the peripheral visual field and therefore more likely that you would miss the gorilla.

The temporal lobe provides information on an object's identity, past experience and possible emotional significance. Using this information, the parietal lobe formulates a plan to react. With the consent of the motor cortex and the prefrontal cortex, the movement plan devised by the parietal lobe is put into action. This is important in sport where you need to visualise successful actions and then react to stimuli quickly and reflexively. In real time, however, you can stall these movements if you get anxious about the consequences of your actions. Think of a sporting situation where you're under pressure: suddenly something you've done thousands of times feels impossible. Maybe you've rehearsed, practised and visualised penalty kicks endlessly, but now your legs feel like lead as you approach the ball. You're thinking about the consequences of missing that World Cup-winning opportunity – or worse still, what if you score? You'll never get a moment's peace again!

How you move will then feed back into your system and influence how you feel. This is significant when it comes to pain. Your muscles getting tense can set some sensory buses off on their pain journey to be interpreted by the stored data. If you have experienced pain while picking up a heavy suitcase in the past, you will place emotional significance on the suitcase: it now represents a threat to your well-being. When you go to pick up a suitcase in the future, the plan of movement devised by the parietal lobe can be a guarded action as you "brace" yourself for the "dangerous" job of picking up this heavy object. If you repeat this again and again, you reinforce guarded movement patterns. You see the suitcase as a potential threat and armour yourself for picking it up, yet the bed you had to lift to get the suitcase out from underneath it was heavier than the suitcase itself and you didn't defend against that in the same way. You've missed the gorilla again.

Very often in persistent pain scenarios you have no idea you are even moving in a guarded way. It has become so ingrained in how you move that it seems normal. I see patients all the time who unknowingly guard their movement or consciously do so thinking it is better for them. The classic case is where I ask a patient to bend down to try and touch their toes and they ask me how I would like them to do it. With a straight back? Bend from the hips? Or curl their spine? Their question tells me that they believe that there is good and bad movement and if they do it one way over another it's somehow wrong. This isn't helpful. It creates an artificial movement. The spine has evolved over millions of years. The moveable bits are there for a reason. I usually tell them to bend down like there's a £50 note on the floor and it's blowing in the wind! That means they usually move fairly quickly and naturally.

There are many situations where you don't even realise that you are making certain muscle movements. This is often likely under times of stress. Grinding your teeth at night; neck and shoulder muscles tightening during a stressful time at work; tapping your foot up and down as you await an important hospital appointment. Some may be obvious, others less so.

The inferior parietal lobe is one of the last regions of the cortex to mature and is influenced by life experience, so it varies greatly among individuals.[22] This is where some facts are stored and retrieved. This area is involved in learning new motor movements and retrieval when imagining an action, adapting to a task and developing a skill. The inferior parietal lobe works with the prefrontal cortex to update your working memory.[23] In the example about lifting a suitcase, if you can update your stored data with new information (lifting the suitcase is not dangerous: you lifted up the bed to reach the suitcase without a problem and the bed is heavier than the suitcase) then you can train the parietal lobe to script new movement patterns through visualisation and motor learning. The amygdala will still try to protect you from the perceived danger associated with lifting, so you will have to negotiate with other parts of your brain by using your updated knowledge and the executive function of the prefrontal cortex to override that guarded response.

As you do this successfully the emotional threat diminishes, and your movements become smoother and less painful. Think of it like learning a new piece on the piano which is different from but sounds similar to another piece you already know. It requires a bit of practice and conscious effort to be able to play the new piece without automatically falling into the old one. Stress can inhibit the ability of the prefrontal cortex to negotiate with other regions of the brain.[24] This can lead to instinctive guarded movements in the presence of a perceived threat. Remember the amygdala can perceive a threat and set the HPA axis in motion before you are consciously aware of it. Having your health hexagon in order will mean you have more space in your stress bucket and more ability to negotiate with your brain to challenge the learned behaviours of guarded motor actions. You can then relearn new motor actions and bypass the pain pathway for that action. It can be done.

Empathy

The **temporal lobe** supports cognitive function, especially language in the dorsolateral region.

Portions of the temporal lobe, prefrontal cortex, cingulate cortex and amygdala make up the social brain, which helps to process incoming sensory stimuli in a social context, including self-awareness and theory of mind.[25] "Theory of mind" is the ability to appreciate the intentions, emotions and beliefs of others. This includes empathy. Theory of mind enables you to compare ongoing events with past events to help predict the outcome of a situation. It can direct your attention to specific signals to help you focus and suppress distracting stimuli. It provides the ability to adopt the perspective of another individual and both empathise with and distinguish yourself from them.

This is why you grimace when you see someone else hurt themselves. The sensory feedback from your facial muscles contorting creates a visceral reaction within your body to help you appreciate the other person's plight, while perhaps also feeling grateful it's not you in pain. Interestingly, studies have shown that those who have had Botox injections for cosmetic reasons are less accurate in interpreting the facial expressions of others, perhaps because they cannot mimic as easily and therefore may not experience that visceral reaction.[26]

In pain terms, when you move in a guarded way the feedback from your muscles will suggest to your pain system that there must be something wrong, and this will feed a pain cycle. If you look at an object that you perceive to be a threat, such as a heavy suitcase, your parietal lobe can come up with a guarded muscle pattern. This guarded action will feed back into your pain system and can get filtered as dangerous, thereby feeding a pain response.

To understand how this works, relax your hand and roll it around in a circular motion. As long as you haven't previously had a significant injury like a fracture, dislocation or surgery, it probably feels normal and effortless. Now make a fist and try that same circular motion. Keep going. Chances are you will start to feel rubbing or crunching in the wrist. You know there is nothing wrong with your wrist, but the guarded movements and tensioning of the muscles are feeding back into the system with a stronger sensory input than when your hand is relaxed. The crunching/rubbing sensation can now be interpreted by your brain as potentially dangerous.

If you do this long enough, you will probably convince yourself you have arthritis. Of course, you don't. Rather, you may be attaching emotional significance to the feedback you get from the muscles – that sensory input, the grinding, the crunching. That emotional significance will depend on your stored data in relation to wrist arthritis. If you have a family member who had problems with their wrist or you rely on your hands to work, there will be a heightened relevance to any potential wrist problem. Your brain's filtering process will use this data to decide how to interpret the sensation.

If you can update your stored data with better information, new evidence that lifting is not dangerous, your brain will start to respond differently and you will be able to move in a different way, resulting in less pain. Bend down like there's £50 blowing in the wind, not with a "fixed" spine.

Body awareness

The **insula** separates the parietal, frontal and temporal lobes and is involved in interoception,[27] which is the emotional awareness of visceral sensations. That includes being aware of your own heartbeat, your own breathing, the feeling in your stomach. The insula is also involved in risk/reward decision-making and contributes to gut instinct. It links body states with emotional awareness. Signals from your senses come together in the posterior insular cortex and are processed to distinguish your own movement from that of others. The anterior insular cortex responds to emotions such as anger, disgust or sexual arousal, and houses a mental image of your own physical state.

Studies have shown that a large subgroup of people with depression have poorer interoceptive awareness of their heartbeat and reduced ability to feel their bodily signals, which may contribute to a sense of lethargy and emotional numbness. People with anxiety, on the other hand, tend to have an acute interoceptive awareness of their bodily signals but they don't necessarily read them properly. They are often very in tune with their body and can feel things that others can't or don't need to. They may misinterpret a small change in heart rate as much greater than it really is, which lends itself to catastrophising and a sense of panic.[28]

The insula and its connections to the amygdala are thought to play an important role in anxiety that can occur with coronary thrombosis.[29] After injury it is very common to become more aware of a body part. You start to notice things you paid no attention to before and interpret them as dangerous. Whiplash is a good example. Following a significant whiplash injury, say as the result of a car accident, you can expect stiffness, reduced range of movement and pain. Because such accidents are typically unexpected, there may be some shock as well as anger and frustration. It may take months before you feel properly recovered (but remember, pain beyond three months is not a reliable indicator of tissue harm or damage).

What then can happen is you start to attribute aches and pains in your neck that you might otherwise never have noticed to the injury. Interoception is drawing your focus to the area. You may have had a very good response to treatment. You may have full range of movement, be sleeping well with no need for medication, be back to all your usual daily activities, including sport. You may even be headbanging to AC/DC without any pain or problem. And then you take a flight across the Atlantic.

You get off the plane and realise your neck is sore. You attribute this to the whiplash injury from months ago. In your mind the only reason you could be in pain is because of the injury. After all, you've flown to the US many times before and it was never a problem. Right? Well, probably you always had some neck ache after an eight-hour flight in economy. It's pretty normal – so normal that you tend to dismiss it. You might be uncomfortable for a day or so but nothing a good night's sleep won't fix, so you don't pay much attention. But following an injury, you become more aware of that body part. You start to notice aches and pains that were always there, but which did not have emotional significance attached to them. Once you've been injured your pain system collects pieces of information in order to protect you for the future, so it draws your attention to any perceived threat. Unfortunately these connections are not always easy to interpret, as you may be starting to understand.

When you have a history of injury, your parking sensors become more vigilant when it comes to that body part and choose to warn you sooner. If you are feeling stressed, tired, angry, frustrated, purposeless or vulnerable, they will warn you even sooner. Under these conditions you have less ability to use your prefrontal cortex to negotiate with your pain system, so the pain lingers and intensifies. But hurt and harm are not the same thing, which is why you need to be able to negotiate with the various aspects of yourself to change this. The frontal lobe helps with that.

Negotiation

The **frontal lobe** makes up one-third of the entire cerebral cortex.[30] It consists of a motor cortex for body control. The **primary motor cortex** is like a map of neurons representing every part of the body. The fingers, lips and tongue have a larger area of representation than the feet and toes, reflecting their dexterity for fine motor movement. Hence a greater portion of the brain is required for these areas. The premotor area is involved in planning, motor learning and the initiation of action. Premotor neurons fire in anticipation or rehearsal of movement. Mirror neurons fire when you observe an action with a specific goal – for instance, watching someone pick something up rather than a random movement without a specific goal. These same neurons will fire when you do the movement yourself. They allow you to learn how to move by watching others. Sports professionals use visualisation to rehearse successful movements, such as hitting the opening drive on a golf course, serving a match-winning point in tennis or scoring a penalty in a World Cup final.

The **supplementary motor cortex** is involved in complex motor movements, in recalling motor programs and in performing unfamiliar tasks, such as learning a new piano piece or changing your golf swing technique. To change your movement behaviour, you have to consciously build new pathways. You might film and then watch your action, helping you to identify how to improve what you are doing. If you want to hit a ball like Rory McIlroy, it helps to watch what he does and attempt to imitate it. (Watching him play piano, however, is unlikely to help your golf swing so be mindful of who you have around you as they may influence your behaviour.)

When you try to relearn a movement, it will feel very alien to begin with. There will be a drop in performance. You will fail many times before you establish new pathways and they become ingrained. If you are used to keeping your back rigid and bending "with a straight back", it will take time to learn to bend down and let your back relax as you do so. You will be slower, you probably won't be able to reach as far and you may feel awkward, vulnerable, frustrated and anxious. Keep your long-term aim to improve in mind and suppress the urge to revert to old methods to avoid short-term disappointment.

When you learn a new skill, the supplementary motor cortex must also inhibit familiar sequences so that you don't fall back into old habits. Ask any sportsperson working on new technique. It requires trust, repetition, patience and a sense of purpose to build new, better pathways. In times of pressure, it's easy to revert to what you know, but that keeps you where you are; it doesn't allow you to move forward. Having your health hexagon in order can make space to keep your long-term view in mind and help you re-route those pathways for the better. To do that, you need to be able to use the highest cognitive function of the brain.

The **prefrontal cortex** is the executive centre of the brain,[31] responsible for cognitive and behavioural functions such as goal setting and self-regulation. It combines your sense of self with past, present and future. The prefrontal cortex juggles a series of operations including reasoning on possible outcomes and feed-back from past experiences.

To achieve a goal, you consider options, make decisions and anticipate the potential outcomes. The ventrolateral prefrontal cortex links a stimulus with an experience. The ventromedial prefrontal cortex provides emotional meaning to that stimulus. The orbitofrontal cortex considers reward and punishment before a response. The dorsolateral prefrontal cortex is responsible for working memory, such as doing a maths problem in your head. You store parts of the problem in your short-term memory as you carry on with another part of the problem. You can recall old information such as a formula to help you reach an answer. The same thing happens with movement, where you have a sense of what you are doing now and what you need to do next. It's all part of the continuous calculations you are doing as you go about your day. If the current available data are insufficient, the ventro-lateral prefrontal cortex can call on additional information from the temporal lobe. Of course, you can only do such calculations with the formulas you have available to you in your stored data. If these stored data aren't up to date and helpful, you'll come up with the same unhelpful responses.

The **orbitofrontal cortex** gets input from the temporal cor-tex, amygdala and hypothalamus, making it the main centre for emotional processing. It then evaluates the emotional priorities of stimuli and selects behavioural responses based on reward and punishment. This region is activated when you are choosing between a small but likely reward (the quick fix) and a large, less likely reward (delayed gratification). In simple terms, that might be having a burger now because you're hungry or choosing a salad because it's better for you in the long run. This area is also involved with anticipated regret and embarrassment.

Projections from the orbitofrontal cortex to the motor cortex control the degree to which your limbic system influences your behaviour. In a top-down negotiation the orbitofrontal cortex can inhibit immediate emotional and impulsive reactions coming from the senses and re-route your behaviour based on the likely probability of a more appropriate reward. This is crucial in persistent pain recalibration or training: you need to have a purpose, a big picture or long-term goal/reward to get you through the desire to avoid short-term discomfort. You have to imagine how good it would be to go for a walk in the woods again in order to take some uncomfortable steps as you rehabilitate a broken ankle.

The TV survival show *The Island with Bear Grylls* demonstrates this concept clearly. In an episode from 2016, contestant Hannah Campbell, a veteran and lower-limb amputee who lost her leg in a mortar attack in Iraq, suffers phantom limb pain as a result of PTSD. Hannah is initially apprehensive about her ability to perform and survive on the island. She is unsure whether her disability will hold her back and fears letting herself and the team down as this is her first major undertaking since her amputation. Very quickly it becomes clear that Hannah is an extremely capable individual, a natural leader and someone her peers rely on for direction and support.

Under Hannah's de facto leadership this diverse group are surviving and thriving in this most challenging experiment. All seems to be going well until one night there is a monumental thunderstorm. Hannah is transported back to Iraq as the violent storm triggers memories of the mortar attack. The sounds of the storm are the sensory stimulus that Hannah's brain recognises as dangerous. This ultimately leads to a severe onset of phantom limb pain. Hannah's experience of the thunderstorm-produced phantom limb pain is a perfect example of a central tenet of this book, that pain beyond three months is not a reliable indicator of tissue damage. In Chapter 3, I also said the nociceptors, those threat-detecting nerve endings that people misinterpret as pain fibres, are neither sufficient nor necessary for a pain experience – also aptly demonstrated in what happened to Hannah. Persistent pain is not simple.

Because pain represents a threat to your well-being, your limbic system attaches emotional relevance to the things you see or activities you do that it perceives to be potentially threatening. When faced with these stimuli, the amygdala will alert you to a "threat". The insula will make you aware of your vulnerable body parts, and the anterior cingulate cortex will prompt you to decide how to react. You need to use your prefrontal cortex to negotiate with these areas, to overcome the influence the limbic system has in overprotecting you. You have to update your stored data to have leverage in your negotiation. You have to be able to call upon evidence from the various centres of your prefrontal cortex to help you negotiate with yourself effectively.

Each element of your health hexagon plays a part in this negotiation. The mental space provides cognitive insight and evidence to use in negotiation. The physical space builds the strength to do so. The emotional space includes an understanding of your personality as well as the people around you who offer support, trust and the confidence to tread the line between order and chaos. The spiritual space dampens your HPA axis and reduces your stress so you can use your prefrontal cortex to negotiate. Sleep and diet reduce inflammation, which makes your nociceptors vigilant.

Putting it all together

This is by no means an exhaustive or comprehensive analysis of the brain's departments, functions and operations. It's a very basic outline to illustrate that your brain has lots of areas with different responsibilities, all of which work together to interact with the world. The brain filters, organises and reacts to sensory stimuli through its ability to process signals into different departments.

In its simplest form: the amygdala looks for potential threat, danger or reward before the cortex is aware of the stimulus you are encountering. The hippocampus looks for a memory reference for that situation to recall from experience. The anterior cingulate cortex considers how to respond based on feedback and experience, makes you conscious of your situation and talks to the basal ganglia to select an appropriate instinctive response or reaction. All this in that split second between thought and action.

The thalamus receives sensory input and directs it to the appropriate brain area. The insula provides body awareness, and the hypothalamus releases hormones to express how you feel externally, such as changes to your heart rate, blood pressure and vasoconstriction, which helps blood flow to parts of the body needed to react. The parietal lobe is involved in scripting motor behaviour, and the temporal lobe interprets social context to try to predict an outcome. The prefrontal cortex analyses reward and punishment and proposes activity over a longer time frame than the reflexive reaction of the anterior cingulate cortex, and constantly updates to regulate the amygdala. The frontal lobe negotiates on the outcome, sets goals, works towards self-regulation and helps execute a reaction.

Stress can inhibit the frontal lobe's ability to negotiate with the limbic system. Different regions of the brain can have stronger or weaker connections as a result of early brain development and how you have used and trained your brain throughout your lifetime. The brain can only filter the signals with the information available to it. You can update that information consciously by being alert to the prospect of a gorilla in the room but also in recognising that you can be a creature of habit. Sometimes these habits work against you and need updating.

With some understanding of how the brain works – and more importantly how you yourself work – you can consciously influence this filtering process and change your situation. You can expose yourself to new information and update your stored data. You can reorganise the information you already have to fine-tune your response and negotiate with old habits that are getting in the way of necessary new behaviour.

Sara had had neck surgery some years previously to remove a tumour. After the operation she was told to be very careful and not to make any sudden movements with her neck. This surgery was obviously a stressful time and understandably she was very careful as she was terrified that she could paralyse herself if she did move suddenly. As a consequence, she became very robotic in her movements and had developed persistent pain. No one had ever told her that some months after her operation it was OK to start moving naturally again. Her surgeon was more interested in the tumour and whether everything had gone according to plan on that front rather than the musculoskeletal element of her problem.

Very often you have the information within your stored data to help you change how you approach a problem. This was the case for Sara – she just needed to reorganise the data she already had to change how she behaved. I asked her whether, during the years since her operation, she had ever made any sudden movements without thinking. Offhand she couldn't think of anything until we discovered that she had slipped badly on the ice a couple of years ago, landing heavily on her backside but also bumping her head in the fall. She was so aware of her bruised behind that her neck was no longer the focus of her pain. Once she understood that her neck had to have moved suddenly in such a fall and that it was OK afterwards, things fell into place for her. A little apprehensively, she started to consciously turn her head. The muscles guarded a bit as you would expect, but with some practice, reassurance and negotiation between her prefrontal cortex and limbic system, things improved. She was able to turn her head more easily to drive and cycle, she started doing dance classes and her pain subsided.

So far, we have explored two of three elements of the pain pathway. We have looked at how stimuli from your surroundings get into the central nervous system and how your brain processes or filters these signals (Chapter 3). We have looked at how the messages transmitted through the sensory bus journey are influenced by inflammation and stress (Chapter 7), and in this chapter we've looked at how the filtering system in your stored data is influenced by habit, association, reflex actions and focus, and how different parts of your brain negotiate to change your instinctive response. Now it's time to look at the third element: how your brain learns. The obvious way to explain this is with tomatoes.

CHAPTER 12

Predicted Data

Tomatoes

As a baby, you learned about colours. Most likely before you could talk, your parents would have pointed at objects in different colours – red, yellow, green and blue. As you got older perhaps they asked you to point at the red thing. Sometimes you pointed at the correct colour and sometimes the wrong one. Eventually you figured out with greater reliability which object was red. This process allowed your brain to build a cortical representation of the piece of information for the colour red. We call these neurotags.[1] These neurones are distributed pieces of information across various departments of the brain that form a circuit and represent something. Your brain now has a neurotag that represents the colour red. Every time you see something red, the sensory information from that object takes a bus into your central nervous system. Your brain filters the information based on experience and anticipated outcomes. The red neurotag is activated and you "see" red.

With time and practice, your red neurotag becomes reliable and robust in different contexts. Your brain also has to create neurotags for each object as well as the overlap between the object and the colour. A baby's developing brain manufactures a million synapses per second;[2] that's a lot of information being processed and connections being established. Slowly red takes on new meanings. It represents stop, danger, hot, the Chinese flag, Liverpool Football

Club, tomatoes. Each of those associations with red has its own neurotag. All these neurotags communicate with each other and use overlapping information to come up with a conclusion.

In time these simple neurotags grow more mass, that is more networks or circuits that they can connect with to give you the information you need. As life goes on and you learn more and update your stored data, you start to make connections between pieces of information. Tomatoes are red; tomatoes are used in salads; salads evoke the Mediterranean; the Mediterranean represents Italy; and Italy means Silvio Berlusconi! Your brain made all these connections by developing independent neurotags for each piece of information and connected them. Not only are neurotags developing greater mass over your lifetime, they are also gaining complexity in that they connect more and more information.[3]

Of course, not all tomatoes are red. If you're a specialist tomato grower, the word "tomato" may be strongly associated with yellow and yellow means chicken; chicken means coward and so on. If you are Heston Blumenthal, maybe tomatoes mean ice cream and another Michelin star. The point is that you will make connections depending on your own experiences and meaning.

What has this got to do with pain?

Pain works in the same way. It learns to connect all the bits of information available to come up with a conclusion, and this evolves as time goes on. In the case of the red tomato, your brain not only relies on the data from your eyes about colour and shape, but it will also use smell and texture to decide whether this is indeed a tomato – and one that you want to eat. That's all before you've even put it in your mouth and stimulated some of your taste sensors. Your brain processes information to update itself all the time but can only do so with the information available to it. If you see a tomato, you think tomato – but maybe it's an optical illusion. Maybe that tomato is a very convincing cake in the shape of a tomato. To be sure of your conclusion, you need to touch it, smell it, taste it. With limited data, you have to make assumptions.

In the early stages of a pain experience, the sensory data the body sends to the brain from a torn ankle ligament are very helpful to warn you that something has happened and there is a potential threat to your well-being. You withdraw your foot from the danger, an action that happens at a reflex level before you are consciously aware of it. However, this now starts the process of building a neurotag. Your brain starts to collect and process information about this situation to protect you for the future.[4] It might do so for instance by telling you that carrying on playing football is dangerous if you've sprained your ankle.

Of course, you already have some knowledge about the potential dangers of football and ankle injuries, but until it happens to you it's just potential. Now that it has happened to you it is real, and your brain's network of information will start to connect the dots. Your brain will recall stories it has heard about others who sprained their ankle. Maybe it's a famous footballer, or your sibling when they were little, or a neighbour from ten years ago. It's all in there and your brain starts to develop and grow that neurotag. Everything that happens from then on will play a part, to a greater or lesser degree, to establish what that neurotag will be affected by. The right or wrong advice on how to deal with that injury will have a major impact.

Now you have a neurotag for ankle pain and this can be activated by different stimuli. These are things that can influence the stimulation of your ankle pain. Some will be more powerful than others. Think of this as the sensitivity of the neurotag. In simple terms when you have a freshly sprained ankle, putting some weight on it and trying to take a step is likely to stimulate the pain. That is peripheralisation of pain. The foot will hurt to move and walk on. As the tissue heals, weight-bearing becomes easier and less likely to stimulate the pain. You can take more steps, walk for longer distances, try hopping or running. The sensitivity of the neurotag to weight-bearing has adjusted, allowing you to do more of it before the neurotag – ankle pain in this instance – gets activated.

While you were recovering in the early stages of the injury, shoes probably made a difference. Wearing a supportive lace-up boot provided some stability; a cushioned trainer made it a little easier to take a step; walking in a hard-soled leather dress shoe was difficult and painful. In time, with further healing, the shoes became less important and the sensitivity of the neurotag to shoes changed. Although the likelihood of either weight-bearing or a shoe activating your ankle pain neurotag has reduced, this doesn't mean your pain can't still be stimulated by a com-bination of these factors. Walking in a leather shoe may be OK and running in a trainer may be OK, but running in a leather shoe could activate the neurotag. Those two factors coming together could be enough to make you reach the threshold of sensitivity of the neurotag activating the pain.

As the neurotag grows in complexity, the number of things connected to it and therefore potentially able to influence it increases. This is neuronal mass. Some stimuli carry more influence than others. This is neuronal precision. Think of these as kingpins: they can activate the neurotag alone in the absence of any other stimuli. Without a kingpin the neurotag can still be activated, but generally by a number of less powerful stimuli all happening at the same time. Let me try to explain this with a group analogy.

Every Monday night after work a group of 12 friends get together in the local village hall for an exercise class. Everyone benefits from the collective spirit as well as the variety of exercises, which each person wouldn't necessarily do on their own. They push themselves as a group in a way that they wouldn't do individually. A couple of members take it in turns to organise the session with different exercise routines for variety. Each member brings their own element to the group. Some add humour, some motivation, some remain quiet but act as an inspiration, some struggle and some thrive.

Think of each member of the group as a modulating factor of the neurotag that is Monday night club. On a typical Monday night, the group turns up and the neurotag is switched on. Not everyone turns up every week but Monday night club still happens – so the neurotag doesn't require the whole group to be present for it to be activated.

Now let's imagine one of the organisers who puts the session together can't make it. This person is clearly an important element of the success of Monday night club, more so than those who don't contribute to the content of the session. Will the neurotag be activated without them? Yes, because there is another person who also organises the sessions. Monday night club can go ahead without one of them.

What if both don't turn up? Will the neurotag get activated now? Possibly, but not definitely. It will take the other members of the group collectively working together to come up with a session in the absence of the two organisers. It won't be the same without them, but it might still go ahead.

What happens if organisers turn up as does everyone else except for one other member? Will Monday night club go ahead? Of course it will; one person doesn't make a difference if the organisers are there, right? Not if that person has the keys to the village hall. Monday night club isn't happening tonight. OK, I accept they could do it outside the hall, but it's not Monday night club in the village hall if it's not in the village hall.

The point is that various modulating factors of the neurotag can contribute, to a greater or lesser extent, to the neurotag being activated or not. In persistent pain terms this means some things will stimulate your pain quite easily; without them, it might take several things colliding together to stimulate the same pain, depending on the specificity and sensitivity of the modulating factors of the neurotag.

Remember we talked about the bucket theory: when you reach your capacity you overflow and that's when you can become symptomatic. Your neurotag has a threshold or capacity to be stimulated. It might be that a specific stimulus, such as loading the dishwasher, is particularly powerful and fills up your bucket quickly. Without it, it takes quite a few smaller stimuli to reach your capacity. And as I'm sure you realise by now, your capacity for anything depends on your health hexagon being in order. If you don't have much capacity on a given day, because you are being stretched in one or more parts of your hexagon, it might not take many small stimuli to stimulate your neurotag. That is why things can be confusing and inconsistent when it comes to persistent pain. Each person has a unique neurotag for their persistent pain,[5] so what activates yours and which stimuli are more powerful than others will be unique to you.

This complexity is why persistent pain often doesn't make

sense. The apparent random nature of the pain being stimulated when you don't expect it leads to a sense of fragility, vulnerability and fear. Inconsistent flare-ups can leave you doing less and less in case you set off the neurotag. The fact that it doesn't make sense is what you can use to change things.

If you are an active rugby player, getting pain from loading the dishwasher doesn't make sense in the context of what you can do physically. The neurotag's strength and irritability will depend not only on its mass and precision but also on neuroplasticity[6] and your ability to change the neurotag's sensitivity with updated learning and actions. Changing the sensitivity of the dishwasher as a modulating factor to your back pain neurotag will require using the available evidence to negotiate. First you recognise the inconsistency of the pain. Then you register that it doesn't make sense. Building the evidence is crucial here: loading the dishwasher is not dangerous when you can play rugby. As much as you might convince yourself that you are "moving wrong" when you bend to the dishwasher, you can use your prefrontal cortex to question the validity of that thinking and then to change it. You can then start to register that the dishwasher itself may not be the primary modulating factor or kingpin in this situation. It may be that a disorganised health hexagon primes you and the dishwasher just happens to be one of many modulating factors that stimulate the back pain neurotag. That's why the dishwasher provokes pain some days and not others. Persistent pain is complicated.

Closure

As you recover from an acute injury with the natural healing process and rehabilitation, you retain the neurotag but it rarely gets switched on. Your ankle has recovered, you have updated your information, and the neurotag is no longer sensitised. This will probably happen within three months and the neurotag is then like a dormant volcano. There, but not interfering.

Sometimes, however, you can fixate on data you encounter along the way, which then continue to stimulate the neurotag even when those data are no longer reliable or necessary. A regular example I have heard in clinic over the years is a client believing that their flat feet are responsible for their ongoing pain after an ankle injury. In reality they always had flat feet (most people do) and it was never a problem before they sprained their ankle. Now that they have had an ankle injury and someone somewhere noted their flat feet or they googled "foot pain" and found results about flat feet, their flat feet now become a fixation. Thus keeping their foot injury neurotag sensitised and becomes part of their belief system about their pain. This piece of information loosely connected to their ankle issue becomes a kingpin.

It's very common after injury to need closure on a problem before you can trust that it's OK, at which point the neurotag reduces its sensitivity to an appropriate level. If you have doubts, the neurotag can remain more irritable than is necessary. When a jockey falls off a horse and dislocates his shoulder, he knows he's going to be out for a while. It's a tough competitive game and one jockey's misfortune is another's opportunity. An injury means not just the pain and frustration of rehab but also the loss of opportunities. Someone else will take your ride while you're injured and if they do a good job, you may not get back on that horse again, even when you are fit. As a result, jockeys are very motivated to get back to work as soon as possible; every single day counts. Being in pain won't stop them from going back to work, but it will play on their mind. However, the pain may not be a reliable indicator of the extent of the injury.

Dealing with such jockeys taught me something about closure on an injury. I used to think that once we had restored their range of movement, improved their strength and often got them doing exercises that were more challenging than anything they had done before their injury, they would be happy. I used to think that once they got back to work and could race again, they would be happy. I assumed that once they rode a winner, they would feel reassured their shoulder was fine. They weren't. Despite good range of movement, sound shoulder stability tests and riding winners, they'd complain that things didn't feel right. They weren't convinced that things were OK, and no amount of reassurance could satisfy them. Only when they fell off a horse and their shoulder stayed in the socket were they happy.

To desensitise the neurotag, these jockeys need to do the thing that they are fearful of, the thing that caused the problem in the first place. If they pass that test, that convinces them they are OK. They could be black and blue from such a fall, but they are delighted their shoulder stayed in the socket, and that bruise will be insignificant. Context is everything: it is a completely different pain experience to what they might have experienced without the stored data of a previous shoulder dislocation. Following a fall where the shoulder stays in the socket, the stored data get updated almost instantly and the neurotag's sensitivity recalibrates.

I cannot advocate falling off a horse to prove you are OK, and most of us won't need that kind of confirmation to get closure on an injury. You do, however, have to work towards the thing that challenges you in order to lose any fear associated with that activity and desensitise the relevant neurotag. Unfortunately, in

211

persistent pain you are likely to do the opposite. You are likely to avoid doing the thing that injured you in the first place as well as – worse still –avoiding doing anything similar. Restricting your activities makes your neurotag more sensitive, not less. You can't bully or ignore the neurotag; you have to negotiate with it. Nudge it, bit by bit, until it's ready to be challenged with a test that recalibrates it. That might be a 50:50 tackle in football, lifting the heavy object, getting back on the horse.

Starting on the wrong course

In the early stages of injury, the pain response is helpful. It's designed to protect you, helping you to avoid harm or seek help. After three months, however, by which time most injuries have healed sufficiently that you can start challenging them, pain is no longer a reliable indicator of tissue harm or damage. That doesn't mean the pain no longer has a function; it's just that it's no longer a reliable indicator of harm. At this stage the neurotag is influenced by many modulating factors such as astrocyte set points, pro-inflammatory lifestyles, stored data content and the filtering and negotiations between these things. The result is a pain experience that is no longer acting reliably to protect you from tissue damage but is trying to grab your attention at some level. The pain is being stimulated or influenced by complex, indirectly related stimuli that are no longer relevant to tissue healing or integrity.

As time goes on, this becomes what is known as nociplastic or persistent pain. The pain is real because the neurotag representing that pain gets activated by these modulating factors, but those modulating factors are no longer reliable when it comes to tissue integrity. The parking sensors become sensitive, warning you sooner and sooner. This can stop you from doing the things that are good for you, the things that would change the sensitivity of those modulating factors, so the pain goes on.

Pain is an output of the human. In other words, pain is what the brain tells you it is. As a human, your brain is unique to you, as is your cortical signature for your pain.[7] Your experiences, your understanding of a situation, your ability to process signals automatically and to negotiate with multiple pieces of information in real time all influence which neurotags get activated and therefore what experience you have. Your lived experience is formulated by sensory data: how something looks, feels, moves, smells and so on. Your brain filters stored data through existing information and pathways and ultimately comes up with predicted data, which is what you expect should happen when you join the dots. The brain then activates the specific neurotag and delivers a pain message to that body part. It gives it a location and a sensation. This is predicted data. That's what humans do, predict our interactions with the world. Phantom limb pain is predicting pain to be in the foot that isn't there. Whichever way you look at it, the pain is very real.

Pain can occur if any or all of the elements of the pain pathway are sufficiently stimulated. Nociceptive fibres (Chapter 3) react to trauma and inflammation, resulting in pain. Astrocyte set points that influence the flow of messages from the sensory system to the brain are lowered by a pro-inflammatory lifestyle, which contributes to the mass and complexity of stored data (Chapter 11). The negotiations that we are talking about in this chapter result in the pain prediction. Beyond three months from the initial injury, this pain experience can be influenced more by stored data than sensory data.

Remember nociceptive stimulation is neither sufficient nor necessary to deliver a pain experience. If you believe that something is dangerous or harmful, you will have a pain experience even if that is no longer correct. Think of the footballer with the sprained ankle. Initially when the ankle was bruised and swollen, kicking a football would of course be painful. His brain naturally concludes, "Don't kick a football." Those data were correct at the time. However, as the tissues healed, the swelling went down and his range of movement normalised, his balance and power and all the other sensory data returned to normal. If at that point his stored data kept saying, "Don't kick a football," and the predicted data said, "If you do, you'll damage something," it will probably hurt if he tries to kick a ball. Just like an optical illusion, your brain can make you "see" or "feel" things differently.

To treat persistent pain, you need to recalibrate the three influencing factors: sensory data, stored data and predicted data. You might need some help to restore the sensory data to normal: for example, range of movement, strength, power, co-ordination. The stored data recalibration is a combination of updating your knowledge and changing your thinking around things that are no longer relevant. Just becoming aware of the association and inconsistencies between these things can generate a significant change in mindset. You may well need some help with that too, and with identifying any more obscure connections that have gained more influence on the pain neurotag than they should. If your health hexagon is balanced and in order, this will help your stress system and inflammatory systems to be less agitated. This helps reduce the sensitivity of your sensory pathway and gives you greater ability to negotiate with the stored data.

As you recalibrate sensory and stored data and you start nudging yourself closer to the things that are good for you which you have been avoiding, the predicted data will change. As you reinforce your learning, you change the neurotag's sensitivity and you become confident that you are not as damaged as you might have believed and that things can get better. When you've been in pain for a long time the complexity of the problem can feel daunting, and you won't necessarily know where to start. The process can move more quickly than it sounds if you can identify some kingpins early.

Making use of what you already know

Marcus came to see me some years ago. Before his initial assessment, he sent me a large file of documents including various letters from doctors, physios, osteopaths, chiropractors and personal trainers and no less than 14 MRI scans of his back, which had taken place over the previous ten years. When he arrived for his appointment, he told me to "release his iliopsoas".

That statement is a red flag to me. It demonstrates that he is fixated on a piece of information being responsible for his pain. I have two degrees in this subject and thousands of hours of experience. Although I know the origin, insertion, innervation and function of the iliopsoas muscle, I'm pretty sure I couldn't feel my own or tell if I needed it "released". Marcus had had his problem for a decade and if "releasing" his iliopsoas was the solution, as he believed had been done numerous times before by other therapists, then he wouldn't be in front of me. I suggested we approach his problem another way.

Marcus was very successful professionally. He was used to having things his way. When it came to his back, he could afford to keep searching for people who would support his view, even if that wasn't always in his best interests. He travelled frequently and often scheduled one-off appointments with specialists around the world who were willing to "release his iliopsoas" if that's what he wanted. Or specialists who would say, "We've found something on your MRI that could be the cause of your pain." As they only had one appointment with him, the simplest thing to do was offer medication for immediate pain relief and leave it at that. There is little point challenging a patient's belief system if you can't then follow it up. This process reinforced his stored data; he was getting similar answers all over the place. The problem was he wasn't getting any better.

His main problem, as he understood it, was that he had a spondylolisthesis. In simple terms this is where one vertebra sits further forward than it should.[8] There are four grades of spondylolisthesis. Grades I and II don't usually cause huge problems and are typically managed successfully with conservative strategies such as physiotherapy. Grades III and IV are more significant and can require surgical intervention. Marcus told me about having to take board meetings lying on the floor as his back had "gone out" or being stretchered off a flight because his back "went". How he couldn't bend backwards because if he did his vertebra would "slip". He had played sport to a high level in his younger days, so fitness was an important part of his identity. He tried to keep fit in the gym but avoided any activity that involved extension of his spine (bending backwards).

Somewhere along the way he had heard the message that any type of extension activity would worsen a spondylolisthesis and should be avoided at all costs. His first MRI scan identified a grade I spondylolisthesis, which was deemed to be responsible for his acute back spasm. As he understood it, his back was fine and then he did something dangerous, and his vertebra slipped out of line. He wasn't quite sure what he did wrong, but he needed to have it put "back in line" to stop the pain. Releasing his iliopsoas was what he believed to be necessary to get things back in line. Over the years he had numerous pain flare-ups and spasms, and various treatments, opinions and MRI scans. He also had periods of no pain whatsoever. To him these pain-free periods were a matter of luck; his back could "go" at any moment, usually at the most inconvenient times when there were important meetings and deals to be done.

When examining him I asked him to bend forward and see how far he could get. He could bend fully forward and had no difficulty in touching his toes. Then I asked him to bend backwards. He said he couldn't. Wouldn't. I gently placed my hands on his shoulders and directed him into extension. He went rigid, turned and pushed me away, clearly terrified that any extension could be catastrophic for him. At this point I said we needed to talk and asked him to sit down. I had to find a way to help him understand that it was OK to move backwards and that his fear wasn't helping him.

"Over the last decade," I said, "you've had 14 MRI scans."

He nodded.

"You've had scans when you've been in pain."

He nodded.

"You've had scans when you've recently been in pain, but your pain had settled."

He agreed.

"You've even had scans just to check if everything was OK."

Again, he nodded.

"In all those years of scans, has it ever been anything other than a grade I spondylolisthesis?"

He shook his head. Never.

"Do you think that if this vertebra was unstable and moving in and out that at least once in 14 MRI scans over ten years in a variety of painful states, it would have been something other than a grade I? At least one time?"

There was a long pause. "I never thought of it that way," he said. "I guess if it was moving, the scans would have shown it."

I reassured him that his spine was stable, and things weren't moving in and out randomly. Why he had pain in the first place I couldn't say, but everything that had happened since, his belief that his spine was unstable and that he should never bend backwards, was causing him to live in fear. The fear was fuelling his pain pathway.

With some apprehension, he allowed me to try bending him backwards again. Gently, he started to move into extension. Little by little, he went further and further. Within 20 minutes he was actively bending backwards. A major piece of unreliable stored data that had been contributing to his pain had now been reorganised, and we never had to go looking for his iliopsoas. He had fallen off the proverbial horse by bending backwards because he used the evidence of the MRI scans in a way he hadn't considered before. His mindset had shifted.

The reality is, he would have been moving into extension numerous times over that last decade, but he wasn't consciously aware of doing so. You often have the evidence you require within your stored data; you just might need help identifying it so you can use it in your negotiation with yourself. If it's not there, you'll need a plan to gather the evidence necessary to help change the sensitivity of the neurotag. Organising your health hexagon will go a long way to giving you more capacity to do so. I suspect Marcus had a spondylolisthesis from his late teens as a result of a pars defect,[9] but he wasn't aware of it until the first MRI was done in his mid-40s. Because he was in pain when the scan was done, the "flaw" found on the MRI was determined to be the source of the pain. The narrative was created and his neurotag continued to receive this message for a decade based on the available stored data: a spondylolisthesis is the cause, don't bend backwards or you'll make it worse.

Lazy labels

In the 1990s magnetic resonance imaging (MRI) was seen as the answer to all back problems. MRI scans offered amazing detail of the spine compared to the basic images previously available with X-rays. Unlike X-rays, MRI showed nerves, soft tissues and the holy grail – the discs. The term "slipped disc" was coined due to the apparent movement of these disc-like structures into the space where only nerves should be. Countless diagnoses of slipped discs were given out and patients who had previously been oblivious to the existence of these omnipotent rascals were now convinced that said discs would forevermore go flying out of their backs and out the window every time they bent over or sneezed. Surgeons became very busy fusing spines to stop discs from moving or replacing them to fill the gap, to varying degrees of success. Thirty-plus years of research into radiologically reported changes on MRI of normal spines has shown us that discs don't move. They do, however, change shape and sometimes they hit nerves, but the individual doesn't necessarily experience pain when this happens. Some do, some don't.

Further evidence that pain is more complicated than meets the eye: the "damaged" disc, which was considered for a while to be the main reason someone would or wouldn't have back pain,

219

is now considered normal if its shape is a bit distorted, especially in the lower vertebrae. Scans of normal spines of asymptomatic people show spondylolisthesis at a rate of about 14 per cent in 50-year-olds.[10] These are people with no pain at all and yet they have a spondylolisthesis. What's seen on a scan isn't always the source of pain,[11] but if you assume it is, then sooner or later it will become a source of pain.[12]

The language used around back pain and many musculo-skeletal pain problems can be unhelpful. There are many lazy labels out there, such as "slipped disc", which give you an erroneous impression about the fragility of your back, and this leads you to feel vulnerable. It stops you from doing the things that are good for you and makes your neurotags sensitive to anything that could present an opportunity to "put your back out of line".

There are loads of these labels, each of which has the power to influence your behaviour subliminally. Sciatica, for example, is not a diagnosis. It's a symptom. Sciatica means referred pain down your leg coming from your back. There are a variety of reasons as to why you could have referred pain into your leg so a catch-all term isn't sufficient to differentiate between causes. It's a bit like saying to someone with a pain in their head that their diagnosis is a headache. That's not very helpful.

Beyond the vagueness, the problem is that people may get conflicting or confusing information about what they should do for their sciatica based on someone else's experience, but they might have a very different diagnosis than that person. It's back to the Gladys effect. You'll believe Gladys because she's a trusted friend instead of an expert who challenges you. Gladys had sciatica so she must know what's she's talking about.

When it comes to something like sciatica, I suggest people think about it like a dog. A poodle is a dog, and so is an Alsatian, but they are very different breeds of dog. Your sciatica may not be the same breed as someone else's sciatica and even if it is, within the same breed there are very different temperaments.[13] Your sciatica may not behave the same way as someone else's. Getting advice from Gladys about how to look after a chihuahua when she has a St. Bernard is not necessarily going to help you much.

Health services are stretched the world over and health care professionals are under pressure to get people in and out as quickly as possible. It's easier to give someone a quick and ambiguous label (a "pulled muscle", a "bad back", "old age", "arthritis", "slipped disc", "RSI", "out of line", "degenerative") without clarifying what they mean by it. It's easier to give a prescription for medicine or exercise or even dismiss someone's pain and send them on their way because as a health care professional you know (rightly) that this person doesn't need scans, injections or surgery. The problem is the patient is going to go away and ask Gladys's opinion or Dr Google and the neurotag is going to love the complexity of that.

Making pain fit – missing the point

When you are in pain you will look to make sense of it. The problem is you can make things fit that shouldn't. A fun website on spurious correlations demonstrates this beautifully.[14] This website displays data charts showing correlations between utterly random things. One example shows that the number of people who died by becoming tangled in their bedsheets correlates with per capita cheese consumption; another that the number of films that Nicolas Cage appears in correlates with the number of people who have drowned by falling into a pool. Your neurotag is looking to make sense of things for your own protection, but it can link things that appear to make sense but don't or no longer need to correlate. When you are dealing with a crisis or prolonged stress, the sensitivity of your pain system heightens. You find yourself in pain, so you try to make it fit. But forcing it to fit makes things worse in the long run as you reinforce belief systems or generate new connections for your neurotag. The real success lies in seeing that the stress event or stressful lifestyle is what's triggering the pain – and that pain does not mean damage.

Over 25 years ago I was knocked off my bicycle by a car. A driver looking the wrong way pulled out of a side road. With no time to stop, I cycled straight into the car, flipped over my bicycle, rolled down the bonnet and ended up under the car's front wheels on the road outside Heuston train station in Dublin at rush hour on a Friday.

Lying under a car in the middle of the road at one of the busiest junctions in Ireland, I recall only silence. I remember the sense of embarrassment. Somehow I thought I'd be blamed even though it wasn't my fault. I could sense that everyone was looking at me, even though all I could see was a tyre and the car's undercarriage. The silence was broken by the bus driver leaning out of his window shouting, "It's her fault, she wasn't looking!" A small consolation, but welcome all the same.

I remember getting out from underneath the car and seeing the driver with her head in her hands, convinced she had killed me. I remember knocking on her window and seeing her startled look of disbelief that I wasn't a police officer ready to cuff her and take her away. I remember her rolling down the window and the beeping of cars as they demanded to get on with their journeys.

I remember repeating again and again, "My bike, my bike." The front wheel was mangled, handlebars contorted and various cables dangling everywhere.

Years later, I realise that she was in shock too and she didn't handle the situation as well as she should have. She got out of her car and just kept saying, "You're OK then. Are you sure you're OK?" Before I knew it, she had driven off, never to be seen again. My bike had been retrieved by a passer-by and was now resting against the wall of the Guinness Brewery. I was left standing on a traffic island; the passing cars, buses and taxis had no idea of what had happened just a few minutes before. I remember my jelly legs hesitating to cross the road to safety as car after car whizzed by.

On and off for more than 20 years I've had neck pain. For many of those years, every time my neck hurt I blamed the driver who wasn't paying attention and nearly killed me. I was angry with her for driving off, for her lack of remorse, for leaving me stranded. I relived those events in my mind. I wished I could have articulated at the time what I needed; that I expected her to fix me, fix my bike, take me home and check in a few days later to see if I was indeed OK.

Every time I got neck pain I searched for answers. How could this still be happening? I was working in a hospital at the time and I convinced junior doctors to refer me for an X-ray as the pain was so bad. MRI scans were uncommon in those days, but had I had the chance, I'd probably have had half a dozen and still been no wiser.

I went through a variety of pillows, stuck needles in my own neck, coaxed my physiotherapy colleagues to manipulate me, electrocute me, squeeze me, stretch me, push me and pull me. Sometimes it helped, sometimes it didn't. Year after year, the neck pain came and went. Meanwhile I was treating plenty of people in pain, and learning more and more about it. Yet despite helping others I couldn't quite help myself. And then I went on holiday and had an epiphany.

Turkey was beautiful. I remember noticing how good my neck felt. That was a relief, as often hotel pillows would leave me awake most of the night and cranky during the day. I had my boys jumping off my shoulders in the swimming pool or sitting on them for long hikes. I allowed myself to lounge around and fall asleep on hard plastic sunbeds. I went to the gym a couple of times and lifted weights and used machines I wouldn't ordinarily use. It all felt fine.

After two weeks we flew home, arriving into Gatwick airport at 3 a.m. I had prebooked airport parking so we could drive in and out without having to search around for tickets or machines to pay. I was so organised I had cleared my inbox on the flight on the way over, deleting the car parking email as the entrance barrier recognised the licence plate and would automatically do so again on the way out. It was all fine until the barrier at the car park wouldn't open and demanded I pay £340 to leave.

I pressed the buzzer to speak to the operator, convinced that this would be easy to sort out and we'd be on our way shortly. No such luck. The guy had no record of the car being prebooked and I had no email to prove it. Thirty minutes later after calling the bank, trying to retrieve a deleted email and circular arguments about prebooking, I was allowed to exit after signing a form to say that if I couldn't prove I had prebooked parking within 24 hours, I would be liable for a charge of roughly £500.

I drove out of that car park and as I reached the roundabout a few hundred metres from the barrier, I felt an intense neck pain.

Burning right across my neck, the back of my head felt like it was stuck in a vice and my shoulder blades belonged to someone else. I smiled. It was a perfect epiphany. This was exactly what I'd been trying to explain to my patients for the last few years.

The stress of this situation, the tiredness, the stupidity, the arguments, the frustration – all of it created a cascade of stress hormones that stimulated my pain centres, and my neck started to guard and spasm. The event created the reaction, and the pain was the outcome. This was the moment that allowed me to recalibrate my response. I would use this example as a way of helping others.

Had I not understood this pain event I could very easily have blamed a million and one things for the pain. The pillows in the hotel, the boys jumping off my shoulders, the flight, the luggage, the hire car, that sandwich I ate on Tuesday. I could have made rational and reasoned arguments for many of them, and I could have built up a host of mechanisms for my neurotag that I would then associate with potential threats, thereby giving my neck more reasons to generate pain in the future. Instead I realised that the pain I was experiencing, the real burning intense pain and limitation of movement, was ultimately because I'd deleted an email (due to my personality trait desire for orderliness) and an argument had ensued.

Knowing this wasn't enough to stop my pain. I needed to find the email for a start, and get confirmation from the car park that I wouldn't be charged. I needed to trust my neck and get it moving and carry on with my regular exercises instead of avoiding them for fear I'd make matters worse. But within three days my neck pain had settled. This could have taken weeks in the past.

It's not always that clear-cut. Often the pain event comes on after the stress event. It might be hours later; it might be months.

What is important to realise is that the pain can act as an alarm to tell you that you are stretched or stressed over something. If you can understand what it's trying to tell you, you can take proactive steps to control and regulate your response. You can look at a flare-up and use it as an opportunity to learn. In that instance I learned not to delete emails until the relevant event was over. I learned that it's no big deal if you have to sign a form that could result in a surcharge when you know you've prepaid. You can sort it out in the morning and get the kids home. I learned there's no point in trying to negotiate with someone who has no power to make a decision. I learned that a problem like that is not really a problem in the grand scheme of things; it's an inconvenience. I learned that there is a learning opportunity in every experience, good and bad. I learned that having my health hexagon in order gave me way more capacity to cope with life's uncertainties and helped me out of a flare-up too. For the first time in probably 15 years, I didn't blame that driver.

Pain is clever, but not wise. It uses the knowledge available to it to come up with a conclusion, and then you feel it. But there is a difference between knowledge and wisdom. Knowledge is knowing that a tomato is a fruit. Wisdom is knowing not to put it in a fruit salad.

CHAPTER 13

Recalibrating Persistent Pain

MY JOB HAS taught me that there is no winner of the game of life. It's the journey that counts and making the most of the situation you find yourself in with the tools at your disposal. How you start that journey is not of your choosing. The circumstances you grow up in, the people who guide or hinder you, the decisions you make, your goals and purpose all shape what you do and who you become along the way.

There will be challenges you might choose to pursue or shy away from. Things can go for you and against you. You must take responsibility for yourself as you are the only one who can live your life. Of course, you'll need help from other people along the way, but you must set the course and be the driver of your own life. You can learn from each situation you find yourself in. Your brain will be processing the information anyway so don't be a passenger. Your conscious acknowledgement of what happens to you can help organise how you process those experiences and how you will respond in the future, so pay attention. What you need to take from any scenario, success or failure, will depend on what you are aiming for.

A privilege of my job is that I see patterns unfold in front of my eyes. My patients teach me so many things. If many different people are showing or telling you the same thing, it's worth paying attention. Over the years I have worked with patients

227

who have had to cope with the worst situations you can think of. Major accidents, degenerative neurological conditions, terminal illness, abuse, bereavement, paralysis, amputation. I have met victims of war, torture and kidnap, and encountered people who have had to make the choice to kill or be killed. I have also dealt with people who are generally seen as having experienced major success. Olympians, world-renowned athletes, hugely successful business owners, the super-rich, decorated academics and more. It is notable that most of them are not necessarily fulfilled by their achievements. Mostly my clients fall somewhere between these extremes. People trying to get through every day, juggling work, family, health, the pressures put on them by society and the pressures they put on themselves.

My job has also taught me that although you might think you know how you would cope with a crisis, you have no idea how you will react until you find yourself in it. All you can do is prepare yourself as best you can to have the capacity to cope with the unexpected. Everyone gets stressed at times; it is an essential component of survival. You might not experience it in an emotional context, but your body will be dealing with it in some way or other.

My work has taught me that the capacity to cope with stressors and what represents a threat is different for everyone. We all have our triggers and tolerances. I have seen people over the years who catastrophise about what I might see as a minor problem, yet they manage major crises with a logical calmness and sense of perspective that I aspire to emulate. Others seem to have tremendous capacity to cope with endless challenges only to find themselves derailed by a seemingly small event.

It's true that "Life is what happens to you when you are busy making other plans",[1] but it's important to have plans all the same. The health hexagon is a way to organise the things you can control to manage stress, to give you the capacity to negotiate for yourself and to navigate towards whatever your destination is. When life throws something at you from left field, the hexagon offers a framework to help you cope.

A patient I had known for many years suddenly lost his much-loved wife in a tragic accident. The trajectory of his life changed in an instant. A couple of days after the accident I saw him out running. He was using his hexagon to get through the day, understanding that some order in the chaos was going to provide a way through disaster.

In this book I have tried to lay out some of the principles I have learned through 25 years of working with people in all circumstances of life. I believe pain plays a role in trying to guide you when you haven't paid attention to other warning signs. Pain lets you know when you are drifting too far into order or chaos. If you only ever see pain as an indicator of damage, then you are missing one of its major functions.

Pain can represent a threat to your well-being. It grabs your attention, forcing you to stop and consider. It is a mentor, a guide to get you back on track. Pain's primary function is to protect you and teach you for the future. Let's say you ski down a mountain and break your leg; you know you'll feel pain, but how you will cope with that scenario is unknown. Maybe you'll discover you don't like the lack of independence that comes with being in a cast for months, and this inspires you to organise your health hexagon as best you can to aim for independence in your old age. Maybe breaking your leg teaches you that you don't have to be in the office every hour of every day. Maybe it teaches you that you need to relinquish some control, which might free up some time to offload and do things that help empty your stress bucket. Maybe breaking your leg isn't as bad as you thought it would be. Maybe you cope better than you thought you would, and that gives you the resilience and confidence to take on new challenges.

I was dealing with a jockey once who fractured his spine. When I was explaining the nature of his injury, he surprised me by saying, "I was so worried what it would be like to break my back, but now that I know what it's like I'm not so worried about it happening again." I must stress that these were stable fractures and relatively minor, but it was striking how he gained a kind of confidence from the injury rather than feeling vulnerable.

If you are 50 and rupture your Achilles tendon playing squash against a 20-year-old, it might be your body trying to tell you something. If you get pain for no good reason, like your back goes tying your shoelaces, it's likely it has been waiting to happen. You need to get your hexagon in order if a basic daily task is enough to cause your bucket to overflow. Maybe your muscles were so tense you didn't even realise you were primed until you went into spasm. Maybe it's time to get some exercise if tying your shoes is your limit. Your pain system is trying to grab your attention to let you know some lifestyle changes are required. Perhaps you have taken more on than you can cope with. You were so buried in the forest of your life that you couldn't see the wood from the trees until pain made you stop. It's a blunt tool but it lets you know when you are far enough off track that you need to recalibrate.

Patients come to see me when they are in pain. No one comes because they are feeling good. It's pain that drives them to seek help. It's pain that forces them to deal with a problem. Without pain there wouldn't necessarily be an incentive to take time out of a busy life and consider what might need changing. When they do come looking for help it is an opportunity to look at their health hexagon more broadly. It is an opportunity to ask: Why are they experiencing persistent pain? What are they fearful of? Why is their body reacting this way? What is their purpose, their direction of travel? What is pain trying to alert them to?

Your pain experience will be influenced by the context the pain occurs in, the perceived threat to your well-being and how your nervous system has been wired and conditioned to respond. With persistent pain, the attitude that pain is caused only by damage leads to a sensitised, more vigilant pain system – and this results in more pain, not less.

Pain can also be used as an excuse to avoid confronting the changes you need to make. Maybe you're in an unhappy relationship or a job you never wanted. Maybe you're afraid to challenge yourself to fulfil your ambitions or explore your potential for fear of judgement or failure. Maybe you are lonely. Maybe you're the one everyone else goes to for help. Pain is still trying to tell you something, and it may get louder until you take notice.

Pain is always real, but it does not always mean you are damaged. It does not mean you are fragile. It does not mean you are broken. It is trying to help you pay attention – but not always for the reasons you expect.

To recalibrate persistent pain, there are several steps to consider. We will start with negotiation – not so much with other people, but with yourself.

Incessant thoughts and toddler tantrums

In his book *Solve for Happy*, Mo Gawdat sets out a simple yet powerful premise. Your thoughts, your inner voice, are not you. Many of us have nagging repetitive thoughts, whether about something being wrong, fear about the future, unhealthy comparison or self-blame. We are inherently designed to look at things negatively to protect us from danger, so this voice of doubt popping up incessantly is almost universally experienced. Gawdat suggests you give this nagging voice of doubt an identity to separate it more clearly from yourself. He calls his Becky, after an irritating school friend who was always negative and annoying. When an incessant thought pops into his head, he stops and says, "Becky, is that really true?" He then gets on with doing something constructive and purposeful, and Becky stops interfering.

I call mine Elvis primarily because of the JXL remix of the Elvis song "A Little Less Conversation".[2] When a recurring negative thought pops into my head, I say, "Elvis, stop. That's not helpful. A little less conversation, a little more action please." I look at what I can do, which part of my health hexagon needs some attention, and I get on with doing something constructive.

I see persistent pain as playing a similar role to Becky or Elvis. Pain is the fire alarm that grabs your attention to protect you from what you are doing or about to do and prompts you to make a decision. Persistent pain doesn't mean damage but you must still take notice and use your health hexagon to prevent the pain from interfering with doing the things that are good for you.

In the *Like Mind, Like Body* podcast,[3,4] Stefanie Reyes explains how thinking about pain as a toddler's toy plastic banana that randomly pops up in unexpected places helped her recalibrate her 20-year history of debilitating persistent pain. After trying everything to fix it, including tests, investigations, scans, treatments, medicines, meditation and all sorts of quackery, she eventually discovered that she could take control of her pain by acknowledging it and recognising that pain did not mean damage or harm; rather it was often a sign that she was anxious or stressed or struggling with some aspect of her life.

When your plastic banana of pain pops up, can you ask yourself: "Does this really make sense?" Does it make sense that I am in pain now doing this thing that I've done a hundred times before without a problem? Does it make sense that loading the dishwasher is painful when I can do a dozen push-ups? Does it make sense to say that my spine is out of line or that I slept "wrong" or that this chair is painful but that one is fine? Your incessant thoughts or your plastic banana or your inner Elvis are trying to tell you something, but what is it they are trying to tell you? Challenge them so they don't dominate everything.

Over the years I have suggested to patients that they view their persistent pain flare-ups like a toddler who is having a tantrum. When a toddler is challenged, they struggle to cope and become upset, frustrated and often irrational. Their behaviour doesn't necessarily make sense. As a parent or guardian, you probably ask yourself some questions, all of which correlate nicely with the health hexagon. Are they tired? That's sleep. Are they hungry? That's diet. Do they need a hug or to vent their frustrations? That's the emotional space. Do they need to burn off some energy or persevere at climbing that piece of play equipment? That's the physical space. Do they need encouragement that they are capable, that they can overcome whatever challenge they're faced with? That's the mental/cognitive space. Do they just need to be a toddler, splashing around in a muddy puddle? That's the spiritual space. When your pain pops up, consider what it is your inner toddler needs and address it like a grown-up.

Pain is there to guide and protect you. When it pops up it's easy to catastrophise and assume the worst, to feel dependent on a magical cure or utterly hopeless. There is plenty you can actually do if you pay attention.

Pain-free moments

I have never met a patient who hasn't had pain-free moments. It may take time to recognise them, but they are there. If you are struggling to identify them, it won't necessarily work to ask yourself, "Am I in pain now?" If your neurotag is hypersensitised, that will probably just switch your pain on. (That in itself demonstrates that your pain is influenced simply by thinking about it and not because you have "moved wrong".)

A better way is to reflect on your day or week and ask yourself, "Do I remember being in pain when I met my friend/watched that show/played that game?" Patients with persistent pain will often say, "Ah, yes, but I was just distracted, that's why I didn't notice the pain." That's often the point – your pain wasn't interfering in that moment. Your pain was turned off. It's not distraction. You were doing something that was good for you, and good for your pain. There will be more and more of those moments if you pay attention. Bank these moments: you will need them when you come to negotiate with your pain system. When you pay attention to what is good for you, it's easier to make yourself do it when you need to but don't want to. Build an arsenal of tools that you can deploy both to prevent pain from building and to use when pain flares.

Does it make sense?

Time and time again patients tell me that they can manage significant physical challenges, such as building a garden fence or running a couple of miles, yet they somehow can't pick the shopping out of the car or climb a flight of stairs. This doesn't make sense. Somewhere along the journey they have fixated on a piece of information that was associated with damage or danger at the time and they've held on to it long after it was relevant. I mentioned paying attention to what's good for you so you can use it when you need to. The opposite is also true when something hurts. Try not to see it as a binary fact, that if something hurts it must be bad. Challenge it. In persistent pain you will hurt when your bucket overflows. The most recent thing you did that stimulated the pain may itself not be bad or dangerous but rather the final drops in the bucket that caused you to overflow. The key is to check whether it makes sense.

Niall, a young footballer, came to see me with two years of knee pain. He initially hurt his knee landing awkwardly after jumping up for a header. He was 17 and had seen several specialists who had repeatedly scanned his knee and couldn't identify anything conclusive. They suggested it was unlikely to be anything serious, but because he was in pain going up and down stairs, they advised he wait until he could manage stairs pain-free before going back to playing football. He didn't need injections or surgeries. He waited and waited and two years later he was still having pain going up and down stairs at home.

This period of Niall's life was an important one for his development from teenager into adulthood and independence. He couldn't do the thing that gave him a sense of identity, that made him feel part of a group, gave him structure, an outlet for frustration, a chance to experience the highs and lows of sport, a social life. The consequences of not playing football "for a bit until things settle" were much more than 90 minutes of running around a couple of times a week.

Despite the lack of signs of anything atypical in his scans and physical assessment, Niall was convinced that his pain showed his knee was unsafe and that if he played football, he would make things worse. We talked about pain-free moments. He had loads: almost everything was painless except the stairs. Every morning the first thing he did was walk downstairs, checking to see if he had somehow magically recovered overnight. He paid close attention to how his knee felt, hoping that today would be the day, but nothing changed.

Next we explored other scenarios where he might encounter stairs. There were plenty. On holiday recently he had stayed in a house by the coast. He didn't recall the stairs being a problem. Why not? "I was swimming in the sea every day and the cold water must have helped. Or maybe the angle of the stairs was different." He regularly ran up and down stairs at school or in the local shopping centre and that was fine. He had even been running for fitness purposes and that was OK too, but the stairs at home had become the thing that stimulated his neurotag. He needed to recalibrate.

He had to keep asking himself that most important question: "Does it make sense? Does it make sense that I can run up and down stairs all over the place but not at home, which is no more dangerous than anywhere else? Does it make sense that I can run, my scan is fine, my physical assessment is fine, but still I should avoid doing the thing I love and the thing that makes me feel part of my friendship group?"

Of course it doesn't make sense. He needed some evidence to help him get back to training, back to doing what he had wanted to do every day for the last two years. He needed to identify those pain-free moments, bank them and use them to negotiate for the confidence to aim for a return to football. He did – and he got back to playing football in a matter of weeks. It wasn't painless initially, but it wasn't dangerous either. The more he nudged his fitness, the better and better his knee felt.

Observe

Pay attention to how you feel and behave when you do certain activities. How do you feel when you exercise, eat healthily, get a good night's sleep, have a project that you are enthusiastic about, share time with friends, have something to look forward to? Notice when you find yourself snapping at someone you love. Then notice how, if you go for a run, you find it easier to laugh, you have more tolerance for situations that might otherwise frustrate you. Notice how you really don't want to go to fit club on a Monday night but when you are walking home, you feel good about having done it. Notice how playing piano or singing or doing a puzzle or painting a picture leaves you feeling more relaxed. Pay attention to the best time to fit these things into your week so that you and those around you get the maximum benefit. Recognise that they are just as important as any other part of your health hexagon and don't compromise on them.

Decompress

Pay attention to how long it takes you to switch off and relax. If you have a commute, can you use it to help you unwind? Read a book, listen to a podcast or just be. If you work from home, can you create a transition that allows you to switch from work mode and into family mode? Go for a walk or a run, shoot some hoops, cut the lawn. Explain to your family why you are going straight out for a run before you engage with them. When you come back, notice whether you now have the capacity to be present.

I once heard a story about members of the band U2 who bought the Clarence Hotel in Dublin so they could stay in it for a couple of weeks after they came back from a world tour. Apparently Bono's wife suggested it, saying that there was no point in coming home a couple of days after playing to a sell-out stadium in São Paulo and expecting to be able to do the school run the next morning. He needed a couple of weeks to decompress, to stop being Bono and start being Dad and Paul Hewson. We can all learn from that.

Downtime

Pay attention to what you need to feel properly refreshed by a break or holiday. Some people benefit most from a series of long weekends, others need two weeks off to truly unwind. Sitting by the pool for a fortnight can be paradise for one person and torture for another. If you know you need something to help you empty that stress bucket, but your family prefer something different, negotiate some of that time for yourself. Maybe you need a couple of days hiking in the mountains before you can lounge around on the beach. Perhaps you could go off and do that on your own or with a like-minded friend for a few days at some stage in the year. If you explain your reasons and how everyone truly benefits from this, it is possible to make it work. Perhaps you also need to be able to check in with your work while you are on holiday, but you need to figure out enough for you and those around you.

Your life is the entirety of your hexagon. Work is part of that, but not all of it. The purpose of having a break is to have a change of scene, of perspective, the chance to take off a mask or try on a different one. You might need to put rules in place to help you make this happen.

If you don't get the rest you need or you are working more than is good for you, it's highly likely your pain will flare up. You might blame the pillow or the mattress or the flight, but it's probably none of those things.

Read the signposts

If you find yourself feeling unsettled, consider why that might be. Is there someone you find difficult to deal with? Why is that? What can you do about it? How can you change your perspective on the situation? I know patients who purposely avoid having meetings with certain people on a Friday afternoon. They understand that these people fill their stress bucket, and they are not going to go into their weekend overflowing. That is not avoiding a problem; it's smart management of themselves and their circumstances based on insight.

Maybe you don't like confrontation but your job requires it. You are going to need space in your stress bucket for that if you want to carry on. You need to get better at managing confrontation safely or it will eat at you. You can do things that are difficult and challenging for you, but you need enough space to do them. Pay attention to what gives you that space and when best to deploy it. Do you need to go to the gym in the morning to feel calm or do you need to go to the gym in the evening to punch something? Maybe what you need is a regular coffee with a friend, mentor or peer to offload. Pay attention to what works for you so that you don't overflow. If you don't read the signs, pain will step in.

Who are you impressing?

Many patients I see are trying to live up to other people's ideals or expectations. They often then feel disappointed or rejected when they don't get the acknowledgement they crave for their perceived achievements. Ask yourself why you are doing something and who you are trying to please. Are you doing it for recognition from someone else or because it's moving you in the direction you want to go? If along the way other people appreciate what you are doing, which makes you feel supported, motivated or vindicated, that's great. But if you are doing something specifically to be acknowledged in those ways, you might be setting yourself up for disappointment.

My wife is an interventionalist cardiologist. One evening at dinner one of our boys said: "Mum, how many lives did you save today?" "Actually, son, I saved two lives today," she replied. "Great," he said. "What did you do with the rest of your day?"

I think that's perfect. No matter how well you think you are doing, someone else is always going to set the bar higher.

I see many young parents in my clinic who are trying to juggle busy lives and are aiming for perfection in every area, from work to kids to fitness to social life and more. No one is perfect at everything all the time. Good is good enough in most areas of your life so that you don't miss what is important in other areas.

You can be your own worst enemy sometimes. My patient Mark once drove home from the north of Spain after a couple of weeks away. It was late evening when he arrived back and the logical thing to do was unpack the bags, maybe put a wash on, have a cup of tea and an early night. Instead, Mark went out and spent two hours tackling the garden, cutting the grass and raking up leaves in the fading light. A pain flare-up inevitably followed, and not because of the drive home or the beds on holiday or anything else. It was because he didn't have enough capacity for the garden on top of the drive, and he overflowed into pain. Sometimes you have to know when you've done enough.

Quantity

Pay attention to how much is enough *for you*. Many things you do will both fill and empty your bucket. Some exercise is good; too much will add more than it bails. Work is good; too much is not. Sleep is good, but long weekend lie-ins may not work for you. Diet is important, but obsessing about what you eat isn't helpful. Switching off helps, but cropping out isn't necessarily in your best interests. You need people in your life, but you need time to be yourself also. Pay attention to when you don't have enough to do and how that feels as well as to when you take on too much, so you don't repeat the mistake in the future. It's OK to say, "I don't have the capacity for that right now," or negotiate what you can delegate if you are going to take it on.

It sounds like a lot of work, but so much of it will take care of itself if you have a purpose, if you know what you are aiming for. If you want to be in less pain and as independent as you can be in your 80s and 90s, then set some structure now around your sleep, diet and exercise. That's half of it taken care of already. I regularly ask myself whether my 80-year-old self will thank me for the way I'm living today.

What do you expect?

My wife had a patient in her 80s with heart failure, who was assessed as suitable for a biventricular pacemaker. When Eleanor first presented at the clinic, she couldn't walk the length of the room. She was so weak and out of breath she struggled to get from her wheelchair to the examination couch. Six weeks after the procedure, Eleanor came back for a follow-up in the outpatients department. My wife happened to see her en route, walking across the car park, through the hospital and down the corridor to the waiting area. What a transformation! This was why she did her job.

Fully expecting a positive response, my wife asked her patient: "So how are you doing?"

"Oh doctor, I'm no better."

Her heart sank. "But you look so much healthier and you walked the whole length of the hospital. Six weeks ago, you were struggling to get out of the chair."

"But I used to be able to climb mountains and go for hikes when I was in my 40s."

There it was, the curse of the unrealistic expectation.

I hear people say "I used to be …" time and time again. I used to be fitter, I used to be thinner, I used to be more important. Persistent pain often gets fuelled by a loss of identity. You can stay grieving the loss of your former abilities, or you can enable yourself to do something else. My patients inspire me constantly, reimagining their goals after catastrophic injury or illness. A direction of travel is essential: with that in mind, you can move little by little forwards from wherever it is you are now. You may be able to get back to where you were or beyond, depending on what you are dealing with, but you have to enable yourself to move towards your destination. Magical thinking won't do it.

Set your expectations of yourself too high and you might feel dejected and disappointed. This will activate your HPA axis, inflammatory system and pain pathway. Set them too low, and it will probably have the same effect. I believe it's important to always be aiming for something just outside your reach. That way you always have a purpose, something to work towards.

Let it go

Placebo is a powerful tool. The placebo effect is now well recognised as having significant therapeutic benefits across a variety of conditions and symptoms.[5] Studies have even shown that you can train the body to respond to a placebo even when you know it is a placebo. Kidney transplant patients, who need to take powerful immunosuppressant drugs, can condition their body to require less of the active drug by introducing a placebo drug alongside associated stimuli.[6] The idea is that if you take the active medicines and a placebo with, say, a strong smell or taste or while listening to a distinctive piece of music, you train the body to associate these external stimuli with the response of the active drug. Over time you reduce the dose of the active drug while keeping the associated stimuli and get the same biochemical effects as if you were taking the full dose of the active drug.[7]

Placebo response has also been shown to be higher in patients with anxiety disorders.[8,9] This may explain in part why some patients with persistent pain jump around from one thing to another, getting a short-lived positive response each time before the effect wears off. Because they get some good short-term relief from each new intervention, they believe that there must be a magic cure out there which they just need to find. The answer is more likely to lie in treating their anxiety and recalibrating their health hexagon.

Just as placebo is powerful, so too is its opposite, nocebo: a negative response to a stimulus. I have talked a lot here about trying to avoid associating actions, activities or objects with danger. It is important to decondition your response to such things if they have become a nocebo. Equally you don't want to turn a placebo into a nocebo. People with persistent neck pain often have a favourite pillow. They may put a lot of time, energy and money into finding the right pillow and they are very strongly attached to it. Why that particular pillow works is probably quite complicated and maybe many other things in their life have played a role, but the importance of that pillow is now an essential element of their narrative.

What happens when that pillow is not there? Perhaps you're staying with a friend or away for work. The lack of your pillow now becomes a nocebo, which heightens the pain response, leading to a bad night's sleep and further galvanising the narrative that there is only one pillow that works for you. I like my pillow but I have trained myself not to attach unnecessary significance to its importance for the quality of my sleep. There are many things we do out of conditioning, superstition, habit or comfort. If these things help you balance your health hexagon, great, but don't let them become a burden when they don't need to be. Do you really need to be foam rolling your IT band? Do you genuinely need your spine realigned every couple of weeks? Do you need a hot pack or an ice pack *every* night?

Don't force things to fit. Many patients try endlessly to justify why something hurts that doesn't make sense or why something worked that doesn't make sense. It's impressive how convincing we can be when we desperately want something to be true. If you find yourself trying to justify why something hurt this time but not every time, pause and ask, "Does this make sense?" That's all you need to know. Paying attention to when it doesn't hurt or when you do something equally or more challenging that doesn't hurt allows you to see that it doesn't fit. When you find yourself trying to justify a belief with phrases like, "It's because I bent and twisted," or "I didn't warm up properly," or "We Smiths all have bad backs," challenge their validity. They can become self-fulfilling prophecies if you are not careful.

Nudge it

If you have identified that something doesn't make sense about your pain, you might think that the solution is to force yourself to do something, to push through the pain to act. No pain, no gain and all that. It won't work. Most likely you will need to recalibrate the sensitivity of the pain pathway. To do this you need to find your baseline for that activity and then nudge it. Don't bully it; that won't work.

Instead, try to identify a kingpin that activates your pain – a big piece of evidence that can help you reorganise the filtering process in your stored data. Something such as, you've had 14 MRI scans and they've shown your spine isn't moving in and out so it's OK to try bending backwards. This can change ingrained behaviour almost overnight. That will work for some elements of the problem, but a sensitised pain pathway will also need retraining from baseline up.

To nudge and retrain your pain pathway you first need to find your baseline. This might be that your hip pain kicks in after 1 km of walking. You've identified that you can manage 5,000 steps around the house, up and down stairs and around the garden without any problem, but going for a walk triggers your pain. You've acknowledged that this doesn't make sense: 5,000 steps adds up to more than a kilometre, so walking 1 km can't be dangerous for your hip.

To nudge yourself from your baseline, you go for a 1 km walk while reassuring yourself that it isn't dangerous. You have an internal conversation with your own thoughts. You remind yourself of the evidence that it isn't dangerous. You pay attention to your surroundings – the trees in blossom or the birds in the sky or the architecture around you – and your senses so you can focus on something besides your hip. Maybe you listen to a podcast or walk with a friend. You get to 1 km and realise that it's not as painful as usual. You register that it's OK. It's safe. You repeat this as frequently as you have the space to add that walk into your bucket, but you do need to be consistent. You notice you feel less sore, less irritable. You are turning up each time to do your walk whether you feel like it or not. You are creating order. The 1 km walk stops representing a threat. It becomes manageable. Now it is no longer a challenge.

Next you nudge. Perhaps 1 km becomes 1.25 km or 1.5 km, or wherever the baseline has shifted to, and you go through the same process, never forcing it but teasing it out consistently. As you see that you can change the sensitivity of your pain, you start to pay attention to what helps you feel OK with further nudges. You notice when your baseline moves along. As your confidence grows, you set yourself a new direction of travel. That might be a Couch to 5K challenge, a well-researched training programme to take you from never running to being able to run 5 km non-stop in nine weeks.[10] This won't happen within a week or two of nudging from your baseline of 1 km: that's not nudging, that's forcing. Instead it might be that when you are consistently walking 8 km or 10 km confidently and without pain, you'll have the evidence to say, "If I can walk 10 km, I can jog for 60 seconds eight times," as per week one of the C25K programme. Reaching the end of the C25K programme is proof that you have recalibrated your sensitivity to 1 km of walking and beyond. That's your equivalent of the jockey falling off his horse and not dislocating his shoulder.

What will you do when the crisis comes?

There will be pain flare-ups along the way – that's inevitable when dealing with persistent pain. When you perceive a threat to your well-being – whether physical, psychological or emotional – your autonomic nervous system goes into a state of defence, and this primes your pain system to respond.

You may not see yourself as someone who gets stressed or you may feel you cope well with certain stressful situations, but everyone has their triggers. Triggers can leave you in a defensive, vigilant state, priming your pain system to react more aggressively to additional minor stresses. This can cause a pain flare-up, even if you have been doing well for some time. Flare-ups can be demoralising, especially if you had been working hard and thought you were on the road to recovery.

All is not lost, however. Flare-ups are an opportunity to question what your pain is trying to tell you and which triggers are contributing to that flare-up. Perhaps you've stopped doing some of the things that are good for you because you were feeling good and didn't think you needed them or didn't have the time. Perhaps you were spending too much time in one part of your health hexagon. Perhaps you've defaulted to old habits and beliefs. Maybe something came at you from left field or your routine wasn't robust enough to allow for a subtle degree of flexibility. Maybe you were putting yourself under more pressure than necessary to achieve more and more. Maybe your hexagon isn't as well organised as it needs to be.

The good thing about a pain flare-up when you are working on your health hexagon is that it will usually settle quicker than it has in the past. It will settle quicker as you interrogate its validity, as you continue to do the things that you know are good for you. Perhaps you just need to go through an exercise routine you used to find difficult when you were struggling with pain but which you have managed to do consistently for weeks. By going through the routine, you give your body the evidence that if it can do that on a good day and a bad day, then you're not broken. That might be all it takes to get back on track. You gain confidence that you can handle the unexpected flare. You'll become less afraid of it.

Your baseline might revert a little and you might have to build back up again, but you'll likely find you build up quicker than before and that will improve your confidence further, desensitise the pain a bit more and reduce the chances of subsequent flare-ups. What form that takes will vary from person to person. Maybe you have to go back to walking instead of running, but the important thing is not to catastrophise. Keep moving when you know the pain doesn't make sense, when there is no justifiable mechanism of injury. Dip into the other parts of your hexagon; rummage around in your tool bag to find something that will keep you moving in the right direction.

Outside of a flare-up, patients often find it useful to spend some time with their pain, to train themselves to avoid fighting it. If your pain has flared up because your defence system is primed, entering a fight with your pain is only going to stimulate your sympathetic nervous system and heighten the pain experience. Try lying down in a safe, neutral environment and focusing on your pain, talking to it or using breathing techniques to calm and regulate your autonomic system. This is known as somatic tracking and can be a powerful way of recognising that you can have some control over the pain. Notice how thinking about your pain makes you feel anxious or apprehensive that you are going to go into some sort of spasm. This can help you see that pain is a neural wiring response: there is a connection between thinking about your pain and the fear it produces in the absence of trauma or a "dangerous" physical movement.

Exploring your relationship with pain and how it can over-power you is healthy. Learning that sometimes you can negotiate with and control it is powerful. In somatic tracking it is not unusual to move the pain around your body, a bit like the plastic banana popping up in places where it doesn't make sense.

It is not "all in your mind"

"Is this pain real?" is one of the most common questions I hear from patients when they start exploring whether their pain makes sense. I hope it's clear by now that the pain is real. It is a real feel-ing with a location. The pain is generated by a nervous system and biochemistry designed to protect you. Pain is your alarm system and it is designed to protect you from harm, whether external or inside you. Pain is your guide, your lookout scout. It analyses risk, weighing all the things you see and don't see like an invisible agent focused on keeping you safe. Pain is your personal SWAT team, helping you navigate danger. Pain learns – and therein lies both the problem and the solution to persistent pain.

The pain is absolutely not "all in the mind", but you will need to use your mind to figure out how much time you need to spend in each part of your hexagon and what needs organis-ing and maintaining in each space. Just because you mow the lawn once, it doesn't stay that way forever. You will have to keep things in order and adapt as life changes. When you get this right, you have capacity to take on new challenges. When you get this wrong, pain will let you know. The pain is not in your head – but the solution is.

My primary message to you is that – excluding serious illnesses such as cancer and acute illness or injury – persistent pain that lasts for more than three months is no longer a reliable indicator of tissue harm or damage. If you have seen the doctors, had the tests and scans, tried various treatments (possibly even including surgery) and searched for magic fixes to no avail, I am confident that getting your health hexagon in order will make the difference.

If I have not yet managed to convince you that stress and a pro-inflammatory lifestyle play a role in stimulating pain, that taking care of your sleep and diet as well as your physical, emotional, spiritual and mental well-being will influence any pain you have, then all I ask is that you pay attention to your own story. Look for the inconsistencies in your narrative. Ask yourself, "Does my pain really make sense?" Start there. Pain will mentor you the rest of the way.

Acknowledgements

On the 23rd of March 2020 when the UK went into the first COVID-19 lockdown, I needed to create some order in the chaos. My way of dealing with a crisis is to come out the other end with something meaningful. Evidence of time well spent. I took a scrap of paper and scribbled on it the things I wanted to achieve professionally in lockdown. First on that list was "write the book". I've had this book or some version of it floating around in my head and gnawing at me for years. Lockdown was an opportunity to put some structures in place towards that purpose. Aiming at completing a book is one thing. Making it happen is something else. Something that requires the help and support of many people. I would like to acknowledge just a few of those people here, but many more have offered support and encouragement along the way, often unbeknown to them, in simple necessary things or words of encouragement, and I thank you all for that.

First and foremost, to my wife, Pegah, for helping me believe that this was a worthwhile project. I am so lucky to share my journey with you. To my boys, Darragh and Daniel, for inspiring me, teaching me and providing joy beyond measure. To all three for working on our hexagons together. To Olivia Bays, my developmental editor, who took a chaotic, rambling first draft and turned it into a coherent piece of work. To Nskvsky for an incredible cover design from minimal instructions. You captured the essence of the book in a single image. To Vikum Liyanaarachchi for the illustrations. To Christina Roth in South Carolina my

251

copy editor who fine-tuned my numerous grammatical mistakes and made my voice clearer than it's ever been. To Marie Doherty for typesetting and Meg Humphries for proofreading so the book you hold in your hands or on your e-reader flows and feels as it should. To my wonderful colleagues Fiona West and Charles Smith for providing the stability required to work on the book alongside my clinical practice. Finally, to all the patients throughout my career who have allowed me the privilege of being part of their lives and entrusting me with helping them navigate the complexities of pain.

Source Notes

Introduction

1. Fayaz, A., P. Croft, R. M. Langford, L. J. Donaldson, and G. T. Jones. "Prevalence of Chronic Pain in the UK: A Systematic Review and Meta-Analysis of Population Studies". *BMJ Open* 6, no. 6 (1 June 2016): e010364. https://doi.org/10.1136/bmjopen-2015-010364.

2. Mills, Sarah E. E., Karen P. Nicolson, and Blair H. Smith. "Chronic Pain: A Review of Its Epidemiology and Associated Factors in Population-Based Studies". *British Journal of Anaesthesia* 123, no. 2 (August 2019): e273–83. https://doi.org/10.1016/j.bja.2019.03.023.

Chapter 1 Purpose of Pain

1. Treede, Rolf-Detlef, Winfried Rief, Antonia Barke, Qasim Aziz, Michael I. Bennett, Rafael Benoliel, Milton Cohen, et al. "A Classification of Chronic Pain for ICD-11". *Pain* 156, no. 6 (June 2015): 1003–7. https://doi.org/10.1097/j.pain.0000000000000160.

2. Asher, Anne. "Persistent Pain Is the New Chronic Pain". *Verywell Health*, last modified 30 August 2022. https://www.verywellhealth.com/persistent-pain-297140.

Chapter 2 Context of Pain

1. Zamorano, Anna M., Inmaculada Riquelme, Boris Kleber, Eckart Altenmüller, Samar M. Hatem, and Pedro Montoya. "Pain Sensitivity and Tactile Spatial Acuity Are Altered in Healthy Musicians as in Chronic Pain Patients". *Frontiers in Human Neuroscience* 8 (2015). https://www.frontiersin.org/articles/10.3389/fnhum.2014.01016.

Chapter 3 The Sensory Bus Ride

1. Huang, Yi-Ming, Ya-Ju Chang, and Chung Hsun Hsieh. "Nerve Conduction Velocity Investigation in Athletes with Trained Lower Extremity for Well-Controlling Movement". *ISBS – Conference Proceedings Archive*, 2005. https://ojs.ub.uni-konstanz.de/cpa/article/view/1122.

2. Jahn, Reinhard. "How Neurons Talk to Each Other". Max-Planck-Gesellschaft, 21 September 2016. https://www.mpg.de/10743509/how-neurons-talk-to-each-other.

3. Herculano-Houzel, Suzana. "The Human Brain in Numbers: A Linearly Scaled-up Primate Brain". *Frontiers in Human Neuroscience* 3 (9 November 2009): 31. https://doi.org/10.3389/neuro.09.031.2009.
4. "Nerve Conduction Velocity". In *Wikipedia*. Last modified 12 January 2023. https://en.wikipedia.org/w/index.php?title=Nerve_conduction_velocity&oldid=1133262745.
5. Laursen, Willem J., Evan O. Anderson, Lydia J. Hoffstaetter, Sviatoslav N. Bagriantsev, and Elena O. Gracheva. "Species-Specific Temperature Sensitivity of TRPA1". *Temperature* 2, no. 2 (11 February 2015): 214–26. https://doi.org/10.1080/23328940.2014.1000702.
6. Tominaga, Makoto. "[Molecular mechanisms of thermosensation]". *Folia Pharmacologica Japonica* 124, no. 4 (October 2004): 219–27. https://doi.org/10.1254/fpj.124.219.
7. Kidd, B. L., and L. A. Urban. "Mechanisms of Inflammatory Pain". *British Journal of Anaesthesia* 87, no. 1 (1 July 2001): 3–11. https://doi.org/10.1093/bja/87.1.3.
8. Latremoliere, Alban, and Clifford J. Woolf. "Central Sensitization: A Generator of Pain Hypersensitivity by Central Neural Plasticity". *Journal of Pain* 10, no. 9 (September 2009): 895–926. https://doi.org/10.1016/j.jpain.2009.06.012.
9. Latremoliere and Woolf. "Central Sensitization", 895–926.
10. Nees, Frauke, Martin Löffler, Katrin Usai, and Herta Flor. "Hypothalamic-Pituitary-Adrenal Axis Feedback Sensitivity in Different States of Back Pain". *Psychoneuroendocrinology* 101 (March 2019): 60–66. https://doi.org/10.1016/j.psyneuen.2018.10.026.
11. Ji, Ru-Rong, Christopher R. Donnelly, and Maiken Nedergaard. "Astrocytes in Chronic Pain and Itch". *Nature Reviews Neuroscience* 20, no. 11 (November 2019): 667–85. https://doi.org/10.1038/s41583-019-0218-1.
12. Tang, James, Mercedes Bair, and Giannina Descalzi. "Reactive Astrocytes: Critical Players in the Development of Chronic Pain". *Frontiers in Psychiatry* 12 (2021). https://www.frontiersin.org/articles/10.3389/fpsyt.2021.682056.
13. "Pathogen Associated Molecular Pattern – an Overview". ScienceDirect Topics. https://www.sciencedirect.com/topics/medicine-and-dentistry/pathogen-associated-molecular-pattern.
14. Kato, Jungo, and Camilla I. Svensson. "Role of Extracellular Damage-Associated Molecular Pattern Molecules (DAMPs) as Mediators of Persistent Pain". *Progress in Molecular Biology and Translational Science* 131 (2015): 251–79. https://doi.org/10.1016/bs.pmbts.2014.11.014.
15. Bianchi, Marco E. "DAMPs, PAMPs and Alarmins: All We Need to Know about Danger". *Journal of Leukocyte Biology* 81, no. 1 (2007): 1–5. https://doi.org/10.1189/jlb.0306164.

16. Neigh, Gretchen N. Manjakh Bekhbat, and Sydney A. Rowson. "Neuroimmunology: Behavioral Effects". *Oxford Research Encyclopedia of Neuroscience*, 24 January 2018. https://doi.org/10.1093/acrefore/9780190264086.013.7.

17. Chawla, Jasvinder. "Low Back Pain and Sciatica: Overview, Pathophysiology, Characteristics of Pain-Sensitive Structures". 22 August 2018. https://emedicine.medscape.com/article/1144130-overview#a1.

18. Latremoliere and Woolf. "Central Sensitization", 895–926.

Chapter 4 How To Think About Balance

1. Syed, Matthew. *Rebel Ideas: The Power of Thinking Differently*. London: John Murray Publishers, 2020, 212–217, https://www.matthewsyed.co.uk/book/rebel-ideas-the-power-of-diverse-thinking/.

2. "Law of conservation of energy," Energy Education, accessed February 2023, https://energyeducation.ca/encyclopedia/Law_of_conservation_of_energy.

Chapter 5 The Physical Space

1. Harber, V. J., and J. R. Sutton. "Endorphins and Exercise". *Sports Medicine (Auckland, N.Z.)* 1, no. 2 (1984): 154–71. https://doi.org/10.2165/00007256-198401020-00004.

2. Nieman, David C., and Laurel M. Wentz. "The Compelling Link between Physical Activity and the Body's Defense System". *Journal of Sport and Health Science* 8, no. 3 (May 2019): 201–217. https://doi.org/10.1016/j.jshs.2018.09.009.

3. Lin, Tzu-Wei, and Yu-Min Kuo. "Exercise Benefits Brain Function: The Monoamine Connection". *Brain Sciences* 3, no. 1 (11 January 2013): 39–53. https://doi.org/10.3390/brainsci3010039.

4. Gordon, Rebecca, and Saul Bloxham. "A Systematic Review of the Effects of Exercise and Physical Activity on Non-Specific Chronic Low Back Pain". *Healthcare* 4, no. 2 (25 April 2016): 22. https://doi.org/10.3390/healthcare4020022.

5. *Fishpeople, A Film about Lives Transformed by the Sea*. Directed by Keith Malloy. Patagonia, 2017. https://www.imdb.com/title/tt12030516/?ref_=tt_mv_close.

6. Noakes, Timothy David. "Fatigue Is a Brain-Derived Emotion That Regulates the Exercise Behavior to Ensure the Protection of Whole Body Homeostasis". *Frontiers in Physiology* 3 (11 April 2012): 82. https://doi.org/10.3389/fphys.2012.00082.

7. Pedersen, B. K., and B. Saltin. "Exercise as Medicine – Evidence for Prescribing Exercise as Therapy in 26 Different Chronic Diseases". *Scandinavian Journal of Medicine & Science in Sports* 25, no. S3 (2015): 1–72. https://doi.org/10.1111/sms.12581.

8. Keller, Gary, and Jay Papasan. *The One Thing: The Surprisingly Simple Truth behind Extraordinary Results*. London: John Murray Publishers, 2013, 187–188.

Chapter 6 The Mental Space

1. Spalding, Kirsty L., Olaf Bergmann, Kanar Alkass, Samuel Bernard, Mehran Salehpour, Hagen B. Huttner, Emil Boström, et al. "Dynamics of Hippocampal Neurogenesis in Adult Humans". *Cell* 153, no. 6 (June 2013): 1219–27. https://doi.org/10.1016/j.cell.2013.05.002.
2. "6 Types of Exercises That Increase Neurogenesis Urology of Virginia". 9 September 2019. https://www.urologyofva.net/articles/category/healthy-living/3640314/10/13/2019/6-types-of-exercises-that-increase-neurogenesis.
3. Ddrobotec. "Why Your Brain Needs Physical Exercise". 17 March 2020. https://ddrobotec.com/why-your-brain-needs-physical-exercise/.
4. Lambourne, Kate, and Phillip Tomporowski. "The Effect of Exercise-Induced Arousal on Cognitive Task Performance: A Meta-Regression Analysis". *Brain Research* 1341 (1 April 2010): 12–24. https://doi.org/10.1016/j.brainres.2010.03.091.
5. Hari, Johann. "Everything You Think You Know About Addiction Is Wrong". TED Talk, 2016. https://www.youtube.com/watch?v=PY9DcIMGxMs.
6. "Do You Believe These 6 Productivity Myths?" *The ONE Thing* (blog), 13 February 2017. https://the1thing.com/do-you-believe-these-6-productivity-myths/.
7. Keller, Gary, and Jay Papasan. *The One Thing: The Surprisingly Simple Truth Behind Extraordinary Results*. London: John Murray Publishers, 2013, 47–48.
8. Matthews, Gail. "The Impact of Commitment, Accountability, and Written Goals on Goal Achievement". *Psychology | Faculty Presentations* 3 (2007). https://scholar.dominican.edu/cgi/viewcontent.cgi?article=1002&context=psychology-faculty-conference-presentations.
9. "02 Why We Need Change: Scotland's Health". In *Public Health Priorities for Scotland*. Edinburgh: Scottish Government, June 2018. http://www.gov.scot/publications/scotlands-public-health-priorities/pages/2/.
10. Roberts, Max, Eric N. Reither, and Sojung Lim. 'Contributors to the Black-White Life Expectancy Gap in Washington D.C.' *Scientific Reports* 10, no. 1 (27 August 2020): 13416. https://www.nature.com/articles/s41598-020-70046-6.
11. Marmot, Michael G., and Robert Sapolsky. *Of Baboons and Men: Social Circumstances, Biology, and the Social Gradient in Health. Sociality, Hierarchy, Health: Comparative Biodemography: A Collection of Papers*. Washington, DC: National Academies Press, 2014. https://www.ncbi.nlm.nih.gov/books/NBK242456/.

12. Edwards, Donald H., and Edward A. Kravitz. "Serotonin, Social Status and Aggression". *Current Opinion in Neurobiology* 7, no. 6 (1 December 1997): 812–19. https://doi.org/10.1016/S0959-4388(97)80140-7.

Chapter 7 The Emotional Space

1. "Hypothalamic–Pituitary–Adrenal Axis". In *Wikipedia*. Last modified 23 December 2022. https://en.wikipedia.org/w/index.php?title= Hypothalamic%E2%80%93pituitary%E2%80%93adrenal_axis &oldid=1129026414.

2. Bremner, J. Douglas. "Stress and Brain Atrophy". *CNS & Neurological Disorders Drug Targets* 5, no. 5 (October 2006): 503–12. https://www.ncbi.nlm. nih.gov/pmc/articles/PMC3269810/pdf/nihms340152.pdf

3. Flinn, Mark V., Pablo A. Nepomnaschy, Michael P. Muehlenbein, and Davide Ponzi. "Evolutionary Functions of Early Social Modulation of Hypothalamic-Pituitary-Adrenal Axis Development in Humans". *Neuroscience & Biobehavioral Reviews* 35, no. 7 (1 June 2011): 1611–29. https://doi.org/10.1016/ j.neubiorev.2011.01.005.

4. Liu, D., J. Diorio, B. Tannenbaum, C. Caldji, D. Francis, A. Freedman, S. Sharma, D. Pearson, P. M. Plotsky, and M. J. Meaney. "Maternal Care, Hippocampal Glucocorticoid Receptors, and Hypothalamic-Pituitary-Adrenal Responses to Stress". *Science* 277, no. 5332 (12 September 1997): 1659–62. https://doi.org/10.1126/science.277.5332.1659.

5. Heim, Christine, D. Jeffrey Newport, Robert Bonsall, Andrew H. Miller, and Charles B. Nemeroff. "Altered Pituitary-Adrenal Axis Responses to Provocative Challenge Tests in Adult Survivors of Childhood Abuse". *The American Journal of Psychiatry* 158, no. 4 (2001): 575–81. https://doi.org/10.1176/ appi.ajp.158.4.575.

6. Liu, Meng-Ying, Lu-Lu Wei, Xian-Hui Zhu, Hua-Chen Ding, Xiang-Hu Liu, Huan Li, Yuan-Yuan Li, et al. "Prenatal Stress Modulates HPA Axis Homeostasis of Offspring through Dentate TERT Independently of Glucocorticoids Receptor". *Molecular Psychiatry* 28, no. 3 (March 2023): 1383–95. https://doi.org/10.1038/s41380-022-01898-9.

7. Apter-Levi, Yael, Maayan Pratt, Adam Vakart, Michal Feldman, Orna Zagoory-Sharon, and Ruth Feldman. "Maternal Depression across the First Years of Life Compromises Child Psychosocial Adjustment; Relations to Child HPA-Axis Functioning". *Psychoneuroendocrinology* 64 (February 2016): 47–56. https://doi.org/10.1016/j.psyneuen.2015.11.006.

8. Coplan, J. D., M. W. Andrews, L. A. Rosenblum, M. J. Owens, S. Friedman, J. M. Gorman, and C. B. Nemeroff. "Persistent Elevations of Cerebrospinal Fluid Concentrations of Corticotropin-Releasing Factor in Adult Nonhuman Primates Exposed to Early-Life Stressors: Implications for the

Pathophysiology of Mood and Anxiety Disorders". *Proceedings of the National Academy of Sciences of the United States of America* 93, no. 4 (20 February 1996): 1619–23. https://doi.org/10.1073/pnas.93.4.1619.

9.   Schore, Allan. "The Neurobiology of Insecure Attachments". In *Affect Regulation and the Origin of the Self: The Neurobiology of Emotional Development*, 378. Hillsdale, NJ: Lawrence Erlbaum Associates, 1994.

10. Brady, K. T., and S. C. Sonne. "The Role of Stress in Alcohol Use, Alcoholism Treatment, and Relapse". *Alcohol Research & Health* 23, no. 4 (1999): 263–71. https://pubmed.ncbi.nlm.nih.gov/10890823/.

11. Wills, Thomas Ashby. "Multiple Networks and Substance Use". *Journal of Social and Clinical Psychology* 9, no. 1 (March 1990): 78–90. https://doi.org/10.1521/jscp.1990.9.1.78.

12. Martin, Elizabeth I., Kerry J. Ressler, Elisabeth Binder, and Charles B. Nemeroff. "The Neurobiology of Anxiety Disorders: Brain Imaging, Genetics, and Psychoneuroendocrinology". *Psychiatric Clinics of North America* 32, no. 3 (September 2009): 549–75. https://doi.org/10.1016/j.psc.2009.05.004.

13. "Oxytocin". In *Wikipedia*. Last modified 16 January 2023. https://en.wikipedia.org/w/index.php?title=Oxytocin&oldid=1133982466#Biological_function.

Chapter 8 The Spiritual Space

1.   Van Dam, Nicholas T., Marieke K. van Vugt, David R. Vago, Laura Schmalzl, Clifford D. Saron, Andrew Olendzki, Ted Meissner, et al. "Mind the Hype: A Critical Evaluation and Prescriptive Agenda for Research on Mindfulness and Meditation". *Perspectives on Psychological Science* 13, no. 1 (January 2018): 36–61. https://doi.org/10.1177/1745691617709589.

2.   Ankrom, Sheryl. "Deep Breathing Exercises to Reduce Anxiety". Verywell Mind. Last modified 27 January 2023. https://www.verywellmind.com/abdominal-breathing-2584115.

3.   Busch, Volker, Walter Magerl, Uwe Kern, Joachim Haas, Göran Hajak, and Peter Eichhammer. "The Effect of Deep and Slow Breathing on Pain Perception, Autonomic Activity, and Mood Processing—An Experimental Study". *Pain Medicine* 13, no. 2 (21 September 2011): 215–28. https://doi.org/10.1111/j.1526-4637.2011.01243.x.

4.   Kox, Matthijs, Lucas T. van Eijk, Jelle Zwaag, Joanne van den Wildenberg, Fred C. G. J. Sweep, Johannes G. van der Hoeven, and Peter Pickkers. "Voluntary Activation of the Sympathetic Nervous System and Attenuation of the Innate Immune Response in Humans". *Proceedings of the National Academy of Sciences of the United States of America* 111, no. 20 (20 May 2014): 7379–84. https://doi.org/10.1073/pnas.1322174111.

5. Zwaag, Jelle, Rob ter Horst, Ivana Blaženović, Daniel Stoessel, Jacqueline Ratter, Josephine M. Worseck, Nicolas Schauer, et al. "Involvement of Lactate and Pyruvate in the Anti-Inflammatory Effects Exerted by Voluntary Activation of the Sympathetic Nervous System". *Metabolites* 10, no. 4 (April 2020): 148. https://doi.org/10.3390/metabo10040148.

6. Vassilakopoulos, T., S. Zakynthinos, and C. Roussos. "Strenuous Resistive Breathing Induces Proinflammatory Cytokines and Stimulates the HPA Axis in Humans". *American Journal of Physiology* 277, no. 4 (October 1999): R1013–1019. https://doi.org/10.1152/ajpregu.1999.277.4.R1013.

7. Wim Hof Method. "Influencing the Immune System". YouTube, 5 March 2019, https://www.youtube.com/watch?v=A6jqaALpEFM.

8. Wim Hof Method. "'Brain over Body' Michigan Study". YouTube, 22 November 2018, https://www.youtube.com/watch?v=YficBlvPwWQ.

9. Wim Hof. "Wim Hof Breathing Tutorial by Wim Hof". YouTube, 28 September 2018, https://www.youtube.com/watch?v=nzCaZQqAs9I.

10. Buijze, Geert A., Inger N. Sierevelt, Bas C. J. M. van der Heijden, Marcel G. Dijkgraaf, and Monique H. W. Frings-Dresen. "The Effect of Cold Showering on Health and Work: A Randomized Controlled Trial". *PLoS ONE* 11, no. 9 (15 September 2016): e0161749. https://doi.org/10.1371/journal.pone.0161749.

11. "Pareto Principle - an Overview". ScienceDirect Topics. https://www.sciencedirect.com/topics/engineering/pareto-principle.

12. Root-Bernstein, Robert, Lindsay Allen, Leighanna Beach, Ragini Bhadula, Justin Fast, Chelsea Hosey, Benjamin Kremkow, et al. "Arts Foster Scientific Success: Avocations of Nobel, National Academy, Royal Society, and Sigma Xi Members". *Journal of Psychology of Science and Technology* 1, no. 2 (1 October 2008): 51–63. https://doi.org/10.1891/1939-7054.1.2.51.

13. Ware, Bronnie. "Regrets of the Dying". Accessed 2023. https://bronnieware.com/blog/regrets-of-the-dying/.

Chapter 9 Sleep

1. "Length of Circadian Cycle in Humans". Circadian Sleep Disorders Network. Last modified 20 April 2022. https://www.circadiansleepdisorders.org/info/cycle_length.php.

2. Blume, Christine, Corrado Garbazza, and Manuel Spitschan. "Effects of Light on Human Circadian Rhythms, Sleep and Mood". *Somnologie* 23, no. 3 (2019): 147–56. https://doi.org/10.1007/s11818-019-00215-x.

3. Matthew Walker, *Why We Sleep: The New Science of Sleep and Dreams*. First Published in Great Britain by Allen Lane, 2017.

4. Walker, *Why We Sleep*.

5. Walker, *Why We Sleep*.
6. Chang, Anne-Marie, Daniel Aeschbach, Jeanne F. Duffy, and Charles A. Czeisler. "Evening Use of Light-Emitting eReaders Negatively Affects Sleep, Circadian Timing, and Next-Morning Alertness". *Proceedings of the National Academy of Sciences* 112, no. 4 (27 January 2015): 1232–37. https://doi. org/10.1073/pnas.1418490112.
7. Carter, Ben, Philippa Rees, Lauren Hale, Darsharna Bhattacharjee, and Mandar S. Paradkar. "Association Between Portable Screen-Based Media Device Access or Use and Sleep Outcomes: A Systematic Review and Meta-Analysis". *JAMA Pediatrics* 170, no. 12 (1 December 2016): 1202–8. https:// doi.org/10.1001/jamapediatrics.2016.2341.
8. Manfredini, Roberto, Fabio Fabbian, Rosaria Cappadona, and Pietro Amedeo Modesti. "Daylight Saving Time, Circadian Rhythms, and Cardiovascular Health". *Internal and Emergency Medicine* 13, no. 5 (August 2018): 641–46. https://doi.org/10.1007/s11739-018-1900-4.
9. Chan, Sharon, and Miguel Debono. "Replication of Cortisol Circadian Rhythm: New Advances in Hydrocortisone Replacement Therapy". *Therapeutic Advances in Endocrinology and Metabolism* 1, no. 3 (June 2010): 129–38. https://doi.org/10.1177/2042018810380214.
10. Clow, Angela, Frank Hucklebridge, and Lisa Thorn. "The Cortisol Awakening Response in Context". In *International Review of Neurobiology*, edited by Angela Clow and Lisa Thorn, 93:153–75. Science of Awakening. Academic Press, 2010. https://doi.org/10.1016/S0074-7742(10)93007-9.
11. Bailey, S. L., and M. M. Heitkemper. "Circadian Rhythmicity of Cortisol and Body Temperature: Morningness-Eveningness Effects". *Chronobiology International* 18, no. 2 (March 2001): 249–61. https://doi.org/10.1081/ cbi-100103189.
12. Cunningham, Tony J., Stephen M. Mattingly, Antonio Tlatenchi, Michelle M. Wirth, Sara E. Alger, Elizabeth A. Kensinger, and Jessica D. Payne. "Higher Post-Encoding Cortisol Benefits the Selective Consolidation of Emotional Aspects of Memory". *Neurobiology of Learning and Memory* 180 (April 2021): 107411. https://doi.org/10.1016/j.nlm.2021.107411.
13. Abercrombie, H., N. Speck, and R. Monticelli. "Endogenous Cortisol Elevations Are Related to Memory Facilitation Only in Individuals Who Are Emotionally Aroused". *Psychoneuroendocrinology* 31, no. 2 (February 2006): 187–96. https://doi.org/10.1016/j.psyneuen.2005.06.008.
14. Abercrombie, Heather C., Ned H. Kalin, Marchell E. Thurow, Melissa A. Rosenkranz, and Richard J. Davidson. "Cortisol Variation in Humans Affects Memory for Emotionally Laden and Neutral Information". *Behavioral Neuroscience* 117, no. 3 (June 2003): 505–16. https://doi.org/10.1037/ 0735-7044.117.3.505.

15. lmunoz. "Stress Hormone Hinders Memory Recall". *Cognitive Neuro-science Society* (blog), 24 July 2013. https://www.cogneurosociety.org/cortisol_memory/.

16. McEwen, Bruce S. "Cortisol, Cushing's Syndrome, and a Shrinking Brain—New Evidence for Reversibility". *Journal of Clinical Endocrinology & Metabolism* 87, no. 5 (1 May 2002): 1947–48. https://academic.oup.com/jcem/article/87/5/1947/2846459.

17. Whitworth, Judith A., Paula M. Williamson, George Mangos, and John J. Kelly. "Cardiovascular Consequences of Cortisol Excess". *Vascular Health and Risk Management* 1, no. 4 (December 2005): 291–99. https://www.ncbi.nlm.nih.gov/pmc/articles/PMC1993964.

18. Mollaioli, Daniele, Giacomo Ciocca, Erika Limoncin, Stefania Di Sante, Giovanni Luca Gravina, Eleonora Carosa, Andrea Lenzi, and Emmanuele Angelo Francesco Jannini. "Lifestyles and Sexuality in Men and Women: The Gender Perspective in Sexual Medicine". *Reproductive Biology and Endocrinology* 18, no. 10 (17 February 2020). https://doi.org/10.1186/s12958-019-0557-9.

19. Leproult, R., G. Copinschi, O. Buxton, and E. Van Cauter. "Sleep Loss Results in an Elevation of Cortisol Levels the Next Evening". *Sleep* 20, no. 10 (October 1997): 865–70. https://pubmed.ncbi.nlm.nih.gov/9415946.

20. Starkman, M. N., B. Giordani, S. S. Gebarski, S. Berent, M. A. Schork, and D. E. Schteingart. "Decrease in Cortisol Reverses Human Hippocampal Atrophy Following Treatment of Cushing's Disease". *Biological Psychiatry* 46, no. 12 (15 December 1999): 1595–1602. https://doi.org/10.1016/s0006-3223(99)00203-6.

21. Besedovsky, Luciana, Tanja Lange, and Jan Born. "Sleep and Immune Function". *Pflugers Archiv: European Journal of Physiology* 463, no. 1 (January 2012): 121–37. https://doi.org/10.1007/s00424-011-1044-0.

22. Walker, *Why We Sleep*.

23. Leproult, et al. "Sleep Loss Results in an Elevation of Cortisol Levels the Next Evening", 865–70. https://pubmed.ncbi.nlm.nih.gov/9415946.

24. lmunoz. "Stress Hormone Hinders Memory Recall".

25. Dimitrov, Stoyan Tanja Lange, Cécile Gouttefangeas, Anja T. R. Jensen, Michael Szczepanski, Jannik Lehnnolz, Surjo Soekadar, Hans-Georg Rammensee, Jan Born, and Luciana Besedovsky. "Gα$_s$-Coupled Receptor Signaling and Sleep Regulate Integrin Activation of Human Antigen-Specific T Cells". *Journal of Experimental Medicine* 216, no. 3 (4 March 2019): 517–26. https://doi.org/10.1084/jem.20181169.

26. Irwin, M., A. Mascovich, J. C. Gillin, R. Willoughby, J. Pike, and T. L. Smith. "Partial Sleep Deprivation Reduces Natural Killer Cell Activity in Humans". *Psychosomatic Medicine* 56, no. 6 (1994): 493–98. https://doi.org/10.1097/00006842-199411000-00004.

27. Prather, Aric A., Denise Janicki-Deverts, Martica H. Hall, and Sheldon Cohen. "Behaviorally Assessed Sleep and Susceptibility to the Common Cold". *Sleep* 38, no. 9 (1 September 2015): 1353–59. https://doi.org/10.5665/sleep.4968.

28. Ibarra-Coronado, Elizabeth G., Ana Ma Pantaleón-Martínez, Javier Velazquéz-Moctezuma, Oscar Prospéro-García, Mónica Méndez-Díaz, Mayra Pérez-Tapia, Lenin Pavón, and Jorge Morales-Montor. "The Bidirectional Relationship between Sleep and Immunity against Infections". *Journal of Immunology Research* 2015 (2015): 678164. https://doi.org/10.1155/2015/678164.

29. Walker, *Why We Sleep*.

30. Watkins, L. R., and S. F. Maier. "Immune Regulation of Central Nervous System Functions: From Sickness Responses to Pathological Pain". *Journal of Internal Medicine* 257, no. 2 (February 2005): 139–55. https://doi.org/10.1111/j.1365-2796.2004.01443.x.

31. Smith, Michael T., and Jennifer A. Haythornthwaite. "How Do Sleep Disturbance and Chronic Pain Inter-Relate? Insights from the Longitudinal and Cognitive-Behavioral Clinical Trials Literature". *Sleep Medicine Reviews* 8, no. 2 (April 2004): 119–32. https://doi.org/10.1016/S1087-0792(03)00044-3.

32. CDC Newsroom. "1 in 3 Adults Don't Get Enough Sleep". 1 January 2016. https://www.cdc.gov/media/releases/2016/p0215-enough-sleep.html.

33. Scott, Alexander J., Thomas L. Webb, and Georgina Rowse. "Does Improving Sleep Lead to Better Mental Health? A Protocol for a Meta-Analytic Review of Randomised Controlled Trials". *BMJ Open* 7, no. 9 (September 2017): e016873. https://doi.org/10.1136/bmjopen-2017-016873.

34. Baglioni, Chiara, Gemma Battagliese, Bernd Feige, Kai Spiegelhalder, Christoph Nissen, Ulrich Voderholzer, Caterina Lombardo, and Dieter Riemann. "Insomnia as a Predictor of Depression: A Meta-Analytic Evaluation of Longitudinal Epidemiological Studies". *Journal of Affective Disorders* 135, no. 1–3 (December 2011): 10–19. https://doi.org/10.1016/j.jad.2011.01.011.

35. Babson, Kimberly A., Casey D. Trainor, Matthew T. Feldner, and Heidemarie Blumenthal. "A Test of the Effects of Acute Sleep Deprivation on General and Specific Self-Reported Anxiety and Depressive Symptoms: An Experimental Extension". *Journal of Behavior Therapy and Experimental Psychiatry* 41, no. 3 (1 September 2010): 297–303. https://doi.org/10.1016/j.jbtep.2010.02.008.

36. Hiscock, H., E. Sciberras, F. Mensah, B. Gerner, D. Efron, S. Khano, and F. Oberklaid. "Impact of a Behavioural Sleep Intervention on Symptoms and Sleep in Children with Attention Deficit Hyperactivity Disorder, and Parental Mental Health: Randomised Controlled Trial". *BMJ* 350 (20 January 2015): h68–h68. https://doi.org/10.1136/bmj.h68.

37. Daghlas, Iyas, Jacqueline M. Lane, Richa Saxena, and Céline Vetter. "Genetically Proxied Diurnal Preference, Sleep Timing, and Risk of Major Depressive Disorder". *JAMA Psychiatry* 78, no. 8 (1 August 2021): 903. https://doi.org/10.1001/jamapsychiatry.2021.0959.

38. Caggiari, Gianfilippo, Giuseppe Rocco Talesa, Giuseppe Toro, Eugenio Jannelli, Gaetano Monteleone, and Leonardo Puddu. "What Type of Mattress Should Be Chosen to Avoid Back Pain and Improve Sleep Quality? Review of the Literature". *Journal of Orthopaedics and Traumatology* 22, no. 51 (8 December 2021). https://doi.org/10.1186/s10195-021-00616-5.

39. Lei, Jia-Xing, Peng-Fei Yang, Ai-Ling Yang, Yan-Feng Gong, Peng Shang, and Xi-Chen Yuan. "Ergonomic Consideration in Pillow Height Determinants and Evaluation". *Healthcare* 9, no. 10 (October 2021): 1333. https://doi.org/10.3390/healthcare9101333.

40. "Sleep Movement and Genetics". 23andMe. Accessed October 2022. https://www.23andme.com/topics/wellness/sleep-movement/.

41. Youngstedt, Shawn D., and Christopher E. Kline. "Epidemiology of Exercise and Sleep". *Sleep and Biological Rhythms* 4, no. 3 (August 2006): 215–21. https://doi.org/10.1111/j.1479-8425.2006.00235.x.

42. Youngstedt, Shawn D., Michael L. Perlis, Patrick M. O'Brien, Christopher R. Palmer, Michael T. Smith, Henry J. Orff, and Daniel F. Kripke. "No Association of Sleep with Total Daily Physical Activity in Normal Sleepers". *Physiology & Behavior* 78, no. 3 (March 2003): 395–401. https://doi.org/10.1016/s0031-9384(03)00004-0.

43. Reid, Kathryn J., Kelly Glazer Baron, Brandon Lu, Erik Naylor, Lisa Wolfe, and Phyllis C. Zee. "Aerobic Exercise Improves Self-Reported Sleep and Quality of Life in Older Adults with Insomnia". *Sleep Medicine* 11, no. 9 (October 2010): 934–40. https://doi.org/10.1016/j.sleep.2010.04.014.

44. Iftikhar, Imran H., Christopher E. Kline, and Shawn D. Youngstedt. "Effects of Exercise Training on Sleep Apnea: A Meta-Analysis". *Lung* 192, no. 1 (February 2014): 175–84. https://doi.org/10.1007/s00408-013-9511-3.

45. Kline, Christopher E., E. Patrick Crowley, Gary B. Ewing, James B. Burch, Steven N. Blair, J. Larry Durstine, J. Mark Davis, and Shawn D. Youngstedt. "The Effect of Exercise Training on Obstructive Sleep Apnea and Sleep Quality: A Randomized Controlled Trial". *Sleep* 34, no. 12 (1 December 2011): 1631–40. https://doi.org/10.5665/sleep.1422.

46. Kline, Christopher E., Gary B. Ewing, James B. Burch, Steven N. Blair, J. Larry Durstine, J. Mark Davis, and Shawn D. Youngstedt. "Exercise Training Improves Selected Aspects of Daytime Functioning in Adults with Obstructive Sleep Apnea". *Journal of Clinical Sleep Medicine* 8, no. 4 (15 August 2012): 357–65. https://doi.org/10.5664/jcsm.2022.

47. Chasens, Eileen R., Susan M. Sereika, Terri E. Weaver, and Mary Grace Umlauf. "Daytime Sleepiness, Exercise, and Physical Function in Older Adults". *Journal of Sleep Research* 16, no. 1 (March 2007): 60–65. https://doi.org/10.1111/j.1365-2869.2007.00576.x.
48. Walker, *Why We Sleep*.
49. St-Onge, Marie-Pierre, Amy Roberts, Ari Shechter, and Arindam Roy Choudhury. "Fiber and Saturated Fat Are Associated with Sleep Arousals and Slow Wave Sleep". *Journal of Clinical Sleep Medicine* 12, no. 1 (15 January 2016): 19–24. https://doi.org/10.5664/jcsm.5384.
50. Walker, *Why We Sleep*.

Chapter 10 Diet

1. Bouchard, C., A. Tremblay, J. P. Després, A. Nadeau, P. J. Lupien, G. Thériault, J. Dussault, S. Moorjani, S. Pinault, and G. Fournier. "The Response to Long-Term Overfeeding in Identical Twins". *New England Journal of Medicine* 322, no. 21 (24 May 1990): 1477–82. https://doi.org/10.1056/NEJM199005243222101.
2. "Junk Food Ad Spending Outstrips UK Government Campaigns as Healthcare Costs of Obesity Soar". CNS Media. 13 October 2017. https://www.nutritioninsight.com/news/junk-food-ad-spending-outstrips-uk-government-campaigns-as-healthcare-costs-of-obesity-soar.html.
3. Carabotti, Marilia, Annunziata Scirocco, Maria Antonietta Maselli, and Carola Severi. "The Gut-Brain Axis: Interactions between Enteric Microbiota, Central and Enteric Nervous Systems". *Annals of Gastroenterology* 28, no. 2 (2015): 203–9. https://www.ncbi.nlm.nih.gov/pmc/articles/PMC4367209/.
4. Kelly, John R., Paul J. Kennedy, John F. Cryan, Timothy G. Dinan, Gerard Clarke, and Niall P. Hyland. "Breaking Down the Barriers: The Gut Microbiome, Intestinal Permeability and Stress-Related Psychiatric Disorders". *Frontiers in Cellular Neuroscience* 9 (14 October 2015): 392. https://doi.org/10.3389/fncel.2015.00392.
5. Clapp, Megan, Nadia Aurora, Lindsey Herrera, Manisha Bhatia, Emily Wilen, and Sarah Wakefield. "Gut Microbiota's Effect on Mental Health: The Gut-Brain Axis". *Clinics and Practice* 7, no. 4 (15 September 2017): 987. https://doi.org/10.4081/cp.2017.987.
6. Carpenter, Siri. "That Gut Feeling". https://www.apa.org/monitor/2012/09/gut-feeling. September 2012, Vol 43, No. 8. Print version Page 50.
7. Strandwitz, Philip. "Neurotransmitter Modulation by the Gut Microbiota". *Brain Research* 1693, pt B (15 August 2018): 128–33. https://doi.org/10.1016/j.brainres.2018.03.015.

8. Witkamp, Renger F., and Klaske van Norren. 'Let Thy Food Be Thy Medicine....When Possible'. *European Journal of Pharmacology* 836 (5 October 2018): 102–14. https://doi.org/10.1016/j.ejphar.2018.06.026.

9. Callaway, Ewen. "C-Section Babies Are Missing Key Microbes". *Nature.* 18 September 2019. https://www.nature.com/articles/d41586-019-02807-x.

10. Rath, Linda. "Inflammatory Arthritis and Gut Health". https://www. arthritis.org/health-wellness/about-arthritis/related-conditions/physical-effects/inflammatory-arthritis-and-gut-health.

11. Diabetes UK. "Low-Calorie Diets". https://www.diabetes.org.uk/guide-to-diabetes/enjoy-food/eating-with-diabetes/whats-your-healthy-weight/low-calorie-diets. Last accessed February 2023.

12. Matthews, Charles. San Francisco Chronicle. December 30, 2007. "Just Eat What Your Great-Grandma Ate". Michael Pollan. https://michaelpollan.com/reviews/just-eat-what-your-great-grandma-ate/.

13. Riebl, Shaun K, and Brenda M. Davy. "The Hydration Equation: Update on Water Balance and Cognitive Performance". *ACSM's Health & Fitness Journal* 17, no. 6 (2013): 21–28. https://doi.org/10.1249/FIT.0b013e3182a9570f.

14. Pross, Nathalie, Agnès Demazières, Nicolas Girard, Romain Barnouin, Francine Santoro, Emmanuel Chevillotte, Alexis Klein, and Laurent Le Bellego. "Influence of Progressive Fluid Restriction on Mood and Physiological Markers of Dehydration in Women". *British Journal of Nutrition* 109, no. 2 (28 January 2013): 313–21. https://doi.org/10.1017/S0007114512001080.

15. Hillyer, Matthew, Kavitha Menon, and Rabindarjeet Singh. "The Effects of Dehydration on Skill-Based Performance". *International Journal of Sports Science* 5, no. 3 (2015): 95–107. http://article.sapub.org/10.5923.j.sports.20150503.02.html#Sec4.

16. Popkin, Barry M., Kristen E. D'Anci, and Irwin H. Rosenberg. "Water, Hydration and Health". *Nutrition Reviews* 68, no. 8 (August 2010): 439–58. https://doi.org/10.1111/j.1753-4887.2010.00304.x.

17. "Drinking Water before Meals Helps Dieting, Says Study". BBC News. https://www.bbc.co.uk/news/health-11057891.

18. FrieslandCampina Institute. "The Importance of Hydration". 9 April 2019. https://www.frieslandcampinainstitute.com/news/the-importance-of-hydration/.

19. Raman, Ryan. "Does Coffee Dehydrate You?" https://www.healthline.com/nutrition/does-coffee-dehydrate-you. 11 December 2019.

20. Haupt, Angela. "Drinking Too Much Water (Hyponatremia): What you need to know". Everyday Health. https://www.everydayhealth.com/hyponatremia/guide/. 17 June 2021.

21. Haupt, Angela. "Drinking Too Much Water (Hyponatremia): What you need to know".
22. The European Food Information Council (EUFIC) food facts for health choices. "How Much Water Should You Drink per Day?" https://www.eufic.org/en/healthy-living/article/how-much-water-should-you-drink-per-day. Last updated 26 March 2020.
23. "How Much Water Should You Drink per Day?"
24. Segers, Anneleen, and Inge Depoortere. 'Circadian Clocks in the Digestive System'. *Nature Reviews Gastroenterology & Hepatology* 18, no. 4 (April 2021): 239–51. https://doi.org/10.1038/s41575-020-00401-5.
25. Sharma, Shweta, Hemant Singh, Nabeel Ahmad, Priyanka Mishra, and Archana Tiwari. "The Role of Melatonin in Diabetes: Therapeutic Implications". *Archives of Endocrinology and Metabolism* 59, no. 5 (October 2015): 391–99. https://doi.org/10.1590/2359-3997000000098.
26. Martínez-Lozano, Nuria, Asta Tvarijonaviciute, Rafael Ríos, Isabel Barón, Frank A. J. L. Scheer, and Marta Garaulet. "Late Eating Is Associated with Obesity, Inflammatory Markers and Circadian-Related Disturbances in School-Aged Children". *Nutrients* 12, no. 9 (21 September 2020): 2881. https://doi.org/10.3390/nu12092881.
27. Mulrooney, Lindsey. "Time-Restricted Eating Improves Glucose Control for Patients with Type 2 Diabetes". https://www.ajmc.com/view/time-restricted-eating-improves-glucose-control-for-patients-with-type-2-diabetes. 29 July 2002.
28. Manoogian, Emily N. C., Lisa S. Chow, Pam R. Taub, Blandine Laferrère, and Satchidananda Panda. "Time-Restricted Eating for the Prevention and Management of Metabolic Diseases". *Endocrine Reviews* 43, no. 2 (9 March 2022): 405–36. https://doi.org/10.1210/endrev/bnab027.
29. Wilkinson, Michael J., Emily N.C. Manoogian, Adena Zadourian, Hannah Lo, Savannah Fakhouri, Azarin Shoghi, Xinran Wang, et al. "Ten-Hour Time-Restricted Eating Reduces Weight, Blood Pressure, and Atherogenic Lipids in Patients with Metabolic Syndrome". *Cell Metabolism* 31, no. 1 (January 2020): 92–104.e5. https://doi.org/10.1016/j.cmet.2019.11.004.
30. Putka, Sophie. "Four Ways Fasting May Help Your Brain". Inverse, 16 April 2021. https://www.inverse.com/mind-body/how-fasting-affects-the-mind-and-the-body.
31. Godos, Justyna, Filippo Caraci, Sabrina Castellano, Walter Currenti, Fabio Galvano, Raffaele Ferri, and Giuseppe Grosso. "Association between Dietary Flavonoids Intake and Cognitive Function in an Italian Cohort". *Biomolecules* 10, no. 9 (9 September 2020): 1300. https://doi.org/10.3390/biom10091300.

32. Angelino, Donato, Justyna Godos, Francesca Ghelfi, Maria Tieri, Lucilla Titta, Alessandra Lafranconi, Stefano Marventano, et al. "Fruit and Vegetable Consumption and Health Outcomes: An Umbrella Review of Observational Studies". *International Journal of Food Sciences and Nutrition* 70, no. 6 (February 2019): 652–67. https://doi.org/10.1080/09637486.2019.1571021.

33. Akbaraly, Tasnime N., Eric J. Brunner, Jane E. Ferrie, Michael G. Marmot, Mika Kivimaki, and Archana Singh-Manoux. "Dietary Pattern and Depressive Symptoms in Middle Age". *The British Journal of Psychiatry: The Journal of Mental Science* 195, no. 5 (November 2009): 408–13. https://doi.org/10.1192/bjp.bp.108.058925.

34. Godos, Justyna, Walter Currenti, Donato Angelino, Pedro Mena, Sabrina Castellano, Filippo Caraci, Fabio Galvano, Daniele Del Rio, Raffaele Ferri, and Giuseppe Grosso. "Diet and Mental Health: Review of the Recent Updates on Molecular Mechanisms". *Antioxidants* 9, no. 4 (23 April 2020): 346. https://doi.org/10.3390/antiox9040346.

35. Broughton, P. M., D. G. Bullock, and R. Cramb. "Improving the Quality of Plasma Cholesterol Measurements in Primary Care". *Scandinavian Journal of Clinical and Laboratory Investigation. Supplementum* 198 (1990): 43–48. https://pubmed.ncbi.nlm.nih.gov/2189209/.

36. Grosso, Giuseppe, Justyna Godos, Fabio Galvano, and Edward L. Giovannucci. "Coffee, Caffeine, and Health Outcomes: An Umbrella Review". *Annual Review of Nutrition* 37 (21 August 2017): 131–56. https://doi.org/10.1146/annurev-nutr-071816-064941.

37. Zeevi, David, Tal Korem, Niv Zmora, David Israeli, Daphna Rothschild, Adina Weinberger, Orly Ben-Yacov, et al. "Personalized Nutrition by Prediction of Glycemic Responses". *Cell* 163, no. 5 (19 November 2015): 1079–94. https://doi.org/10.1016/j.cell.2015.11.001.

38. Zeevi, et al. "Personalized Nutrition by Prediction of Glycemic Responses", 1079–94.

39. Thorp, Alicia Ann, Bronwyn A. Kingwell, Parneet Sethi, Louise Hammond, Neville Owen, and David W. Dunstan. "Alternating Bouts of Sitting and Standing Attenuate Postprandial Glucose Responses". *Medicine and Science in Sports and Exercise* 46, no. 11 (November 2014): 2053–61. https://doi.org/10.1249/MSS.0000000000000337.

40. Fennell, Diane. "Standing, Walking Breaks Linked with Lower Blood Sugar Levels All Day". Diabetes Self-Management, 2 September 2016. https://www.diabetesselfmanagement.com/blog/standing-walking-breaks-linked-lower-blood-sugar-levels-day/.

41. Crawford, Charles K., John D. Akins, Emre Vardarli, Anthony S. Wolfe, and Edward F. Coyle. "Prolonged Standing Reduces Fasting Plasma Triglyceride but Does Not Influence Postprandial Metabolism Compared to Prolonged

Sitting". *PLoS ONE* 15, no. 2 (5 February 2020): e0228297. https://doi. org/10.1371/journal.pone.0228297.

42. Cannell, John J., William B. Grant, and Michael F. Holick. "Vitamin D and Inflammation". *Dermato-Endocrinology* 6, no. 1 (2014): e983401. https:// doi.org/10.4161/19381980.2014.983401.

43. Aranow, Cynthia. "Vitamin D and the Immune System". *Journal of Investigative Medicine* 59, no. 6 (August 2011): 881–86. https://doi.org/10.2310/ JIM.0b013e31821b8755.

44. Penckofer, Sue, Joanne Kouba, Mary Byrn, and Carol Estwing Ferrans. "Vitamin D and Depression: Where Is All the Sunshine?" *Issues in Mental Health Nursing* 31, no. 6 (June 2010): 385–93. https://doi.org/10.3109/ 01612840903437657.

45. Bair, Matthew J., Rebecca L. Robinson, Wayne Katon, and Kurt Kroenke. "Depression and Pain Comorbidity: A Literature Review". *Archives of Internal Medicine* 163, no. 20 (10 November 2003): 2433–45. https://doi. org/10.1001/archinte.163.20.2433.

46. Fernstrom, J. D. "Carbohydrate Ingestion and Brain Serotonin Synthesis: Relevance to a Putative Control Loop for Regulating Carbohydrate Ingestion, and Effects of Aspartame Consumption". *Appetite* 11 Suppl 1 (1988): 35–41. https://pubmed.ncbi.nlm.nih.gov/3056265/

47. Wurtman, R. J., and J. J. Wurtman. "Brain Serotonin, Carbohydrate-Craving, Obesity and Depression". *Obesity Research* 3 Suppl 4 (November 1995): 477S–480S. https://doi.org/10.1002/j.1550-8528.1995.tb00215.x.

48. Ellulu, Mohammed S., Ismail Patimah, Huzwah Khaza'ai, Asmah Rahmat, and Yehia Abed. "Obesity and Inflammation: The Linking Mechanism and the Complications". *Archives of Medical Science* 13, no. 4 (June 2017): 851– 63. https://doi.org/10.5114/aoms.2016.58928.

49. Spector, Tim. *The Diet Myth: The Real Science behind What We Eat.* First Published in Great Britain in 2015 by Weidenfeld & Nicolson.

50. "Eat Chocolate - Good News! Dr Michael Mosley Says Chocolate Is Good for You". *Just One Thing - with Michael Mosley.* BBC Radio 4. Accessed 26 January 2023. https://www.bbc.co.uk/programmes/articles/2DwZMX9FbRd2KFZ1 98GCmD4/good-news-dr-michael-mosley-says-chocolate-is-good-for-you.

51. Poole, Robin, Oliver J. Kennedy, Paul Roderick, Jonathan A. Fallowfield, Peter C. Hayes, and Julie Parkes. "Coffee Consumption and Health: Umbrella Review of Meta-Analyses of Multiple Health Outcomes". *BMJ* 359 (22 November 2017): j5024. https://www.bmj.com/content/359/bmj.j5024.

Chapter 11 Stored Data

1. Arnsten, Amy F. T., Murray A. Raskind, Fletcher B. Taylor, and Daniel F. Connor. "The Effects of Stress Exposure on Prefrontal Cortex: Translating

Basic Research into Successful Treatments for Post-Traumatic Stress Disorder". *Neurobiology of Stress*, Stress Resilience, 1 (1 January 2015): 89–99. https://doi.org/10.1016/j.ynstr.2014.10.002.

2. Sheridan, Nicholas, and Prasanna Tadi. "Neuroanatomy, Thalamic Nuclei". In *StatPearls*. Treasure Island (FL): StatPearls Publishing, 2022. http://www.ncbi.nlm.nih.gov/books/NBK549908/.

3. Lanciego, José L., Natasha Luquin, and José A. Obeso. "Functional Neuroanatomy of the Basal Ganglia". *Cold Spring Harbor Perspectives in Medicine* 2, no. 12 (December 2012): a009621. https://doi.org/10.1101/cshperspect. a009621.

4. Dimsdale-Zucker, Halle R., Maureen Ritchey, Arne D. Ekstrom, Andrew P. Yonelinas, and Charan Ranganath. 'CA1 and CA3 Differentially Support Spontaneous Retrieval of Episodic Contexts within Human Hippocampal Subfields'. *Nature Communications* 9, no. 1 (18 January 2018): 294. https://doi.org/10.1038/s41467-017-02752-1.

5. Bartsch, Thorsten, Juliane Döhring, Axel Rohr, Olav Jansen, and Günther Deuschl. "CA1 Neurons in the Human Hippocampus Are Critical for Autobiographical Memory, Mental Time Travel, and Autonoetic Consciousness". *Proceedings of the National Academy of Sciences of the United States of America* 108, no. 42 (10 October 2011): 17562–67. https://doi.org/10.1073/pnas.1110266108.

6. @neurochallenged. "Know Your Brain: Amygdala". https://neuroscientifically challenged.com/posts/know-your-brain-amygdala.

7. Yang, Ying, and Jian-Zhi Wang. "From Structure to Behavior in Basolateral Amygdala-Hippocampus Circuits". *Frontiers in Neural Circuits* 11 (2017). https://www.frontiersin.org/articles/10.3389/fncir.2017.00086.

8. Ohman, Arne, Katrina Carlsson, Daniel Lundqvist, and Martin Ingvar. "On the Unconscious Subcortical Origin of Human Fear". *Physiology & Behavior* 92, no. 1–2 (10 September 2007): 180–85. https://doi.org/10.1016/j.physbeh.2007.05.057.

9. Weidenfeld, Joseph, and Haim Ovadia. "The Role of the Amygdala in Regulating the Hypothalamic-Pituitary-Adrenal Axis". IntechOpen, 5 July 2017. https://www.intechopen.com/chapters/54565.

10. Lee, Spike W. S., and Norbert Schwarz. "Bidirectionality, Mediation, and Moderation of Metaphorical Effects: The Embodiment of Social Suspicion and Fishy Smells". *Journal of Personality and Social Psychology* 103, no. 5 (2012): 737–49. https://doi.org/10.1037/a0029708.

11. Bell, Susan. "The Smell of Suspicion". USC Dornsife, 30 June 2015. http://dornsife.usc.edu/news/stories/2092/the-smell-of-suspicion/.

12. Martin, Elizabeth I., Kerry J. Ressler, Elisabeth Binder, and Charles B. Nemeroff. "The Neurobiology of Anxiety Disorders: Brain Imaging,

Genetics, and Psychoneuroendocrinology". *Psychiatric Clinics of North America* 32, no. 3 (September 2009): 549–75. https://doi.org/10.1016/j.psc.2009. 05.004.

13. Eden, Annuschka Salima, Jan Schreiber, Alfred Anwander, Katharina Keuper, Inga Laeger, Peter Zwanzger, Pienie Zwitserlood, Harald Kugel, and Christian Dobel. "Emotion Regulation and Trait Anxiety Are Predicted by the Microstructure of Fibers between Amygdala and Prefrontal Cortex". *Journal of Neuroscience* 35, no. 15 (15 April 2015): 6020–27. https://doi.org/10.1523/JNEUROSCI.3659-14.2015.

14. Lavin, Claudio, Camilo Melis, Ezequiel Mikulan, Carlos Gelormini, David Huepe, and Agustin Ibanez. "The Anterior Cingulate Cortex: An Integrative Hub for Human Socially-Driven Interactions". *Frontiers in Neuroscience* 7 (2013). https://www.frontiersin.org/articles/10.3389/fnins.2013.00064.

15. Stevens, Francis L., Robin A. Hurley, Katherine H. Taber, Robin A. Hurley, L. Anne Hayman, and Katherine H. Taber. "Anterior Cingulate Cortex: Unique Role in Cognition and Emotion". *The Journal of Neuropsychiatry and Clinical Neurosciences* 23, no. 2 (April 2011): 121–25. https://doi.org/10.1176/jnp.23.2.jnp121.

16. Etkin, Amit, Tobias Egner, Daniel M. Peraza, Eric R. Kandel, and Joy Hirsch. "Resolving Emotional Conflict: A Role for the Rostral Anterior Cingulate Cortex in Modulating Activity in the Amygdala". *Neuron* 51, no. 6 (21 September 2006): 871–82. https://doi.org/10.1016/j.neuron.2006.07.029.

17. Rehman, Amna, and Yasir Al Khalili. "Neuroanatomy, Occipital Lobe". In *StatPearls*. Treasure Island (FL): StatPearls Publishing, 2022. http://www.ncbi.nlm.nih.gov/books/NBK544320/.

18. Simons and Chabris "The Invisible Gorilla: And Other Ways Our Intuitions Deceive Us". http://www.theinvisiblegorilla.com/gorilla_experiment.html. 2010

19. "Parietal Lobe". In *Wikipedia*. Last modified 6 December 2022. https://en.wikipedia.org/w/index.php?title=Parietal_lobe&oldid=1125843523.

20. Bisley, James W., and Michael E. Goldberg. "Attention, Intention, and Priority in the Parietal Lobe". *Annual Review of Neuroscience* 33 (2010): 1–21. https://doi.org/10.1146/annurev-neuro-060909-152823.

21. Cavanna, Andrea E., and Michael R. Trimble. "The Precuneus: A Review of Its Functional Anatomy and Behavioural Correlates". *Brain* 129, no. 3 (1 March 2006): 564–83. https://doi.org/10.1093/brain/awl004.

22. Wang, Mengxing, Jilei Zhang, Guangheng Dong, Hui Zhang, Haifeng Lu, and Xiaoxia Du. "Development of Rostral Inferior Parietal Lobule Area Functional Connectivity from Late Childhood to Early Adulthood". *International Journal of Developmental Neuroscience* 59, no. 1 (June 2017): 31–36. https://doi.org/10.1016/j.ijdevneu.2017.03.001.

23. Numssen, Ole, Danilo Bzlok, and Gesa Hartwigsen. 'Functional Specializa-tion within the Inferior Parietal Lobes across Cognitive Domains'. Edited by Dwight Kravitz and Chris I Baker. *ELife* 10 (2 March 2021): e63591. https://doi.org/10.7554/eLife.63591.

24. Woo, Elizabeth, Lauren H. Sansing, Amy F. T. Arnsten, and Dibyadeep Datta. 'Chronic Stress Weakens Connectivity in the Prefrontal Cortex: Architectural and Molecular Changes'. *Chronic Stress* 5 (1 January 2021): 24705470211029256. https://doi.org/10.1177/24705470211029254.

25. Frith, Chris D. "The Social Brain?" *Philosophical Transactions of the Royal Society B: Biological Sciences* 362, no. 1480 (29 April 2007): 671–78. https://doi.org/10.1098/rstb.2006.2003.

26. Neal, David T., and Tanya L. Chartrand. "Embodied Emotion Perception: Amplifying and Dampening Facial Feedback Modulates Emotion Perception Accuracy". *Social Psychological and Personality Science* 2, no. 6 (21 April 2011): 673–78. https://journals.sagepub.com/doi/10.1177/1948550611406138.

27. Wang, Xingchao, Qiong Wu, Laura Egan, Xiaosi Gu, Pinan Liu, Hong Gu, Yihong Yang, et al. "Anterior Insular Cortex Plays a Critical Role in Intero-ceptive Attention". *ELife* 8 (15 April 2019): e42265. https://doi.org/10.7554/eLife.42265.

28. Robson, David. "Interoception: The Hidden Sense That Shapes Wellbeing". *The Observer*, 15 August 2021, sec. Science. https://www.theguardian.com/science/2021/aug/15/the-hidden-sense-shaping-your-wellbeing-interoception.

29. Critchley, Hugo D., Stefan Wiens, Pia Rotshtein, Arne Ohman, and Ray-mond J. Dolan. "Neural Systems Supporting Interoceptive Awareness". *Nature Neuroscience* 7, no. 2 (February 2004): 189–95. https://doi.org/10.1038/nn1176.

30. Sendić, Gordana. "Frontal Lobe". Kenhub. Last modified 30 November 2022. https://www.kenhub.com/en/library/anatomy/frontal-lobe.

31. Siddiqui, Shazia Veqar, Ushri Chatterjee, Devvarta Kumar, Aleem Sid-diqui, and Nishant Goyal. "Neuropsychology of Prefrontal Cortex". *Indian Journal of Psychiatry* 50, no. 3 (2008): 202–8. https://doi.org/10.4103/0019-5545.43634.

Chapter 12 Predicted Data

1. Tatta, Joe. "What Is a Pain Neurotag?" Integrative Pain Science Institute. https://integrativepainscienceinstitute.com/pain-neurotag/. Accessed 27 Jan-uary 2023.

2. Center on the Developing Child at Harvard University. "Brain Architec-ture". https://developingchild.harvard.edu/science/key-concepts/brain-architecture/. Accessed January 2023.

3. Wallwork, Sarah B., Valeria Bellan, Mark J. Catley, and G. Lorimer Moseley. "Neural Representations and the Cortical Body Matrix: Implications for Sports Medicine and Future Directions". *British Journal of Sports Medicine* 50, no. 16 (August 2016): 990–96. https://doi.org/10.1136/bjsports-2015-095356.

4. Moseley, G. Lorimer, Alberto Gallace, and Charles Spence. "Bodily Illusions in Health and Disease: Physiological and Clinical Perspectives and the Concept of a Cortical 'Body Matrix'". *Neuroscience and Biobehavioral Reviews* 36, no. 1 (January 2012): 34–46. https://doi.org/10.1016/j.neubiorev.2011.03.013.

5. Mayr, Astrid, Pauline Jahn, Anne Stankewitz, Bettina Deak, Anderson Winkler, Viktor Witkovsky, Ozan Eren, Andreas Straube, and Enrico Schulz. "Patients with Chronic Pain Exhibit Individually Unique Cortical Signatures of Pain Encoding". *Human Brain Mapping* 43, no. 5 (1 April 2022): 1676–93. https://doi.org/10.1002/hbm.25750.

6. Nicolelis, Miguel A. L., and Mikhail A. Lebedev. "Principles of Neural Ensemble Physiology Underlying the Operation of Brain–Machine Interfaces". *Nature Reviews Neuroscience* 10, no. 7 (July 2009): 530–40. https://doi.org/10.1038/nrn2653.

7. Mayr, Astrid, Pauline Jahn, Anne Stankewitz, Bettina Deak, Anderson Winkler, Viktor Witkovsky, Ozan Eren, Andreas Straube, and Enrico Schulz. "Patients with Chronic Pain Exhibit Individually Unique Cortical Signatures of Pain Encoding". *Human Brain Mapping* 43, no. 5 (1 April 2022): 1676–93. https://doi.org/10.1002/hbm.25750.

8. "Spondylolysis and Spondylolisthesis". OrthoInfo – AAOS. Last modified August 2020. https://www.orthoinfo.org/en/diseases--conditions/spondylolysis-and-spondylolisthesis/.

9. "Spondylolysis and Spondylolisthesis".

10. Brinjikji, W., P.H. Luetmer, B. Comstock, B.W. Bresnahan, L.E. Chen, R.A. Deyo, S. Halabi, et al. "Systematic Literature Review of Imaging Features of Spinal Degeneration in Asymptomatic Populations". *American Journal of Neuroradiology* 36, no. 4 (April 2015): 811–16. https://doi.org/10.3174/ajnr.A4173.

11. Ingraham, Paul. "MRI and X-Ray Almost Useless for Back Pain". www.PainScience.com, 27 August 2021. https://www.painscience.com/articles/mri-and-x-ray-almost-useless-for-back-pain.php.

12. Webster, Barbara S., Ann Z. Bauer, YoonSun Choi, Manuel Cifuentes, and Glenn S. Pransky. "Iatrogenic Consequences of Early Magnetic Resonance Imaging in Acute, Work-Related, Disabling Low Back Pain". *Spine* 38, no. 22 (15 October 2013): 1939–46. https://doi.org/10.1097/BRS.0b013e3182a42eb6.

13. "Do Dog Breeds Have Personalities? Data on 17,000 Pups Shows Genetic Roots". https://www.inverse.com/article/52299-do-dogs-have-personality-dna-says-yes.

14. Vigen, Tyler https://www.tylervigen.com/spurious-correlations Accessed October 2022.

Chapter 13 Recalibrating Persistent Pain

1. "Life Is What Happens to You While You're Busy Making Other Plans". Quote Investigator, 6 May 2012. https://quoteinvestigator.com/2012/05/06/other-plans/.

2. Junkie XL, Elvis Presley – A Little Less Conversation (Official JXL Remix) https://www.youtube.com/watch?v=Zx1_6F-nCaw 2011.

3. "Like Mind, Like Body". Google Podcasts. https://podcasts.google.com/search/like%20mind%20like%20body.

4. https://www.curablehealth.com/ Cureable Inc. 2023.

5. Newman, Tim. "Is the placebo effect real?". Medical News Today, 7 September 2017. https://www.medicalnewstoday.com/articles/306437.

6. Kirchhof, Julia, Liubov Petrakova, Alexandra Brinkhoff, Sven Benson, Justine Schmidt, Maike Unteroberdörster, Benjamin Wilde, Ted J. Kaptchuk, Oliver Witzke, and Manfred Schedlowski. "Learned Immunosuppressive Placebo Responses in Renal Transplant Patients". *Proceedings of the National Academy of Sciences of the United States of America* 115, no. 16 (17 April 2018): 4223–27. https://doi.org/10.1073/pnas.1720548115.

7. Kresser, Chris. "The Healing Power of the Placebo Effect—with Jo Marchant". RHR. Chris Kresser, 24 March 2016. https://chriskresser.com/the-healing-power-of-the-placebo-effect-with-jo-marchant/.

8. Piercy, M. A., J. J. Sramek, N. M. Kurtz, and N. R. Cutler. "Placebo Response in Anxiety Disorders". *Annals of Pharmacotherapy* 30, no. 9 (September 1996): 1013–19. https://doi.org/10.1177/106002809603000917.

9. Rutherford, Bret R., Veronika S. Bailey, Franklin R. Schneier, Emily Pott, Patrick J. Brown, and Steven P. Roose. "Influence of Study Design on Treatment Response in Anxiety Disorder Clinical Trials". *Depression and Anxiety* 32, no. 12 (December 2015): 944–57. https://doi.org/10.1002/da.22433.

10. National Health Service, UK https://www.nhs.uk/live-well/exercise/running-and-aerobic-exercises/get-running-with-couch-to-5k/. Crown copyright. Last reviewed 2 October 2020.

Notes

Notes

Notes

Notes